Small Animal Dermatology for Technicians and Nurses

Small Animal Dermatology for Technicians and Nurses

Edited by

Kim Horne AAS, CVT, VTS (Dermatology)
University of Minnesota
St. Paul, MN, USA

Marcia Schwassmann DVM, DACVD
Veterinary Dermatology Center
Maitland, FL, USA

Dawn Logas DVM, DACVD
Veterinary Dermatology Center
Maitland, FL, USA

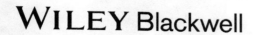

The right of Kim Horne, Marcia Schwassmann and Dawn Logas to be identified as the authors of the editorial material in this work has been asserted in accordance with law.

Registered Office
John Wiley & Sons, Inc., 111 River Street, Hoboken, NJ 07030, USA

Editorial Office
111 River Street, Hoboken, NJ 07030, USA

For details of our global editorial offices, customer services, and more information about Wiley products visit us at www.wiley.com.

Wiley also publishes its books in a variety of electronic formats and by print-on-demand. Some content that appears in standard print versions of this book may not be available in other formats.

Library of Congress Cataloging-in-Publication Data

Names: Horne, Kim (Kim L.), editor. | Schwassmann, Marcia, editor. | Logas, Dawn, editor.
Title: Small animal dermatology for technicians and nurses / edited by Kim Horne, Marcia Schwassmann, Dawn Logas.
Description: Hoboken, NJ : Wiley-Blackwell, 2020. | Includes bibliographical references and index.
Identifiers: LCCN 2019026627 (print) | ISBN 9780470958155 (paperback) | ISBN 9781119108634 (adobe pdf) | ISBN 9781119108627 (epub)
Subjects: LCSH: Veterinary dermatology. | MESH: Skin Diseases–veterinary | Dog Diseases | Cat Diseases | Animal Technicians
Classification: LCC SF901 .S63 2019 (print) | LCC SF901 (ebook) | NLM SF 901 | DDC 636.089/65–dc23
LC record available at https://lccn.loc.gov/2019026627
LC ebook record available at https://lccn.loc.gov/2019026628

Cover Design: Wiley
Cover Images: © Sandy Grable, © Dawn Logas, © Shelley Shopsowitz, © Christie Yamazaki Delan

Set in 10/12pt Warnock by SPi Global, Pondicherry, India

10 9 8 7 6 5 4 3 2 1

To my parents, Jim and Lois Downs, for their love and never-ending support of my career choices. To my husband, Steve Horne, for always being there and making sacrifices that provided me the time needed to follow my dermatology dreams – you are a true partner and best friend. To my work colleagues: Deb Vogt and Pat Berzins, for their supervision and mentoring of leadership qualities; Drs. Pat McKeever, Sheila Torres, and Sandra Koch, for their inspiration and guidance that developed my dermatology passion which allowed me to advance in this profession. And finally to my co-editors, Dr. Marcia Schwassmann and Dr. Dawn Logas – without their willingness to partner on this project, this book would have never happened. Thank you for helping me achieve this, it has been quite the journey!

Kim Horne

To Gail Kunkle who started me on this path. To my co-editors and authors for their patience and good humor in dealing with an obsessive first-time editor. Thank you all!

Marcia Schwassmann

To my husband Paul, my sons Christopher and Jacob, thank you for all your love and support throughout my career. To all the other animals that I have lived with and treated, thank you for making me a better veterinarian.

Dawn Logas

Contents

List of Contributors

Christie Yamazaki Delan DVM
Associate Dermatologist
Animal Dermatology Clinic
Tustin and Ontario, CA, USA

Stephanie B. Duggan AAS, CVT
Animal Care Professional Supervisor &
Dermatology Technician
Veterinary Medical Center
University of Minnesota
St. Paul, MN, USA

Amanda Friedeck BS, LVT, VTS (Dermatology)
Dermatology Technician IV, Medicine
Section Supervisor
Veterinary Medical Teaching Hospital
Texas A&M University
College Station, TX, USA

Sandra Grable AAS, CVT, VTS (Dermatology)
Charter Member
Veterinary Technician III – Dermatology
and Otology
College of Veterinary Medicine
University of Illinois
Urbana, IL, USA

Barbara Haimbach BS, CVT
Dermatology Technician
Hope Veterinary Specialists
Malvern, PA, USA

Kim Horne AAS, CVT, VTS (Dermatology)
Charter Member
Assistant Manager, Small Animal Specialties
and Dermatology Technician
Veterinary Medical Center & Veterinary
Referral Center
University of Minnesota
St. Paul, MN, USA

Dawn Logas DVM
Diplomate of the American College of
Veterinary Dermatology
Veterinary Dermatology Center
Maitland, FL, USA

Marcia Schwassmann DVM
Diplomate of the American College of
Veterinary Dermatology
Veterinary Dermatology Center
Maitland, FL, USA

Shelley Shopsowitz BA, RVT
Small Animal Emergency Technician
Kawartha Veterinary Emergency Clinic
Peterborough, Ontario, Canada

Missy Streicher AAS, CVT, VTS (Dermatology)
Charter Member
Dermatology Technician
College of Veterinary Medicine
Auburn University
Auburn, AL, USA

Jennie Tait AHT, RVT, VTS (Dermatology)
Charter Member
Specialty Services Technician – Dermatology
Yu of Guelph Veterinary Dermatology
Guelph Veterinary Specialty Hospital
Guelph, Ontario, Canada

Preface

Welcome to the 1st edition of *Small Animal Dermatology for Technicians and Nurses.* Veterinary medicine is an ever-changing science, especially when it comes to dermatology treatments. During the writing of this book, revisions were needed since current products were discontinued and new products emerged. At the time of submission, we attempted to include as many existing, relevant products as we could – however, the reader is encouraged to stay up to date with current diagnostic and treatment options as new information becomes available. The authors, editors, and publisher do not necessarily endorse and assume no responsibility for any procedures or products mentioned in this book.

Acknowledgments

The editors would like to thank the publisher for their patience in the long-awaited submission of this book. Many thanks to all the authors and other colleagues for their contributions of chapters and photographs that made this book possible.

Introduction

It seems that the veterinary community can be divided into two groups – those who like dermatology and those that want nothing to do with it! We hope that you are reading this book for your enjoyment; but either way, we recognize that like it or not, small animal dermatology cases are a common occurrence in private practice. These patients often have chronic conditions that are frustrating for the owner as well as the veterinary team.

Our goal with this book is to provide the veterinary technician/veterinary nurse with a solid foundation of knowledge for the most common dermatology conditions. Having the tools to perform dermatology procedures correctly and helpful hints for educating clients will hopefully improve the management of these cases and improve the lives of your dermatology patients.

Kim Horne, AAS, CVT, VTS (Dermatology)
Marcia Schwassmann, DVM, DACVD
Dawn Logas, DVM, DACVD

Section I

The Role of the Veterinary Technician and Nurse

1

Managing the Small Animal Dermatology Patient
Kim Horne

Introduction

The skin is the largest organ of the body and performs many vital functions. It acts as a barrier; offers protection against environmental elements and the development of infections and cutaneous neoplasms; produces vitamin D and keratinized structures such as the hair and claws; regulates temperature; acts as storage for materials such as electrolytes and vitamins; is a primary sense organ; and is an important indicator of general health as well as internal disease (Miller et al. 2013). Skin and ear diseases are very common in our small animal patients. Recent statistics show that pet insurance policyholders' top four medical conditions were related to ear and skin problems (Nationwide 2018). While these may not be the primary reason the patient is presented to the veterinary hospital, clients will often ask to have their pet's skin or ears checked during the visit; or you may discover something during the physical exam that the client was not aware of. Unfortunately, many different dermatological diseases present with similar clinical signs and many of these conditions are only controllable and not curable. Dealing with these cases can be time consuming and frustrating for the pet owner as well as the veterinary staff. The good news is that veterinary technicians and veterinary nurses can play an important role in all aspects of the management of these cases. From taking a complete history, performing diagnostic procedures correctly, to providing thorough client education and following up with the patients' progress – these are the essential elements for achieving success with these cases. The technician's involvement with phone call updates and ensuring recheck appointments are scheduled can improve client compliance and lead to improved patient management.

History

A dermatology history questionnaire can be an efficient way to collect important information. Many dermatology books contain examples of these which can be modified to fit the needs of each practice (Bergvall 2012; Miller et al. 2013). See Figure 1.1 for an example. Filling out the questionnaire will get the client thinking about their pet's dermatology problems, and should be completed prior to the exam. Ideally the questionnaire can be sent to the client in advance of the appointment or the client can arrive early in order to complete the questionnaire. The questionnaire can be very helpful not only for the initial appointment, but also to refer back to if and when the pet's problem recurs or symptoms change.

When taking the history, the breed, age, and sex of the patient can give clues as to

Small Animal Dermatology for Technicians and Nurses, First Edition. Edited by Kim Horne, Marcia Schwassmann and Dawn Logas.

DERMATOLOGY HISTORY

UNIVERSITY OF MINNESOTA
VETERINARY MEDICAL CENTER

1) How long have you owned this pet?_____

2) From what source did you get this pet? _____

_____

3) Is this the first time your pet has had a skin/ear problem?

    ☐ No   ☐ Yes

4) If No, when was the first occurrence? _____

5) What area of the body was involved first? _____

6) What area of the body was involved next?_____

7) Initial appearance of the involved skin? _____

8) How did the involved skin change as time went on? _____

_____

9) What do you think caused the problem? _____

10) Do the parents or siblings have a skin problem?   ☐ No   ☐ Yes   ☐ Unknown

11) Previous medications? _____

12) Response to previous medications?_____

13) Does your pet swim?   ☐ No   ☐Yes

14) What is your pet's bed made of?_____

15) Reason for visit? _____

16) When did this problem begin? _____

17) Is your pet taking any medications currently?   ☐ No   ☐ Yes

    If YES, please list drug and dosage_____

    Response to current meds?_____

18) Any adverse drug or vaccination reaction?☐ No ☐ Yes Describe:_____

19) Any previous illness, surgery or trauma? ☐ No ☐ Yes Describe:_____

20) Any eye or nasal discharge?☐ No ☐ Yes Describe:_____

21) Any vomiting or diarrhea? ☐ No ☐ Yes Describe:_____

22) Any coughing or sneezing?☐ No ☐ Yes Describe:_____

23) Any change in urination or defecation? ☐ No ☐ Yes Describe:_____

24) Any change in food or water intake?☐ No ☐ Yes Describe:_____

25) Any change in weight?☐ No ☐ Yes Describe:_____

26) Current Diets and treats – include amount and frequency: _____

_____

27) Any change in activity or mobility? ☐ No ☐ Yes Describe:_____

28) Any skin or hair coat concerns?☐ No ☐ Yes Describe:_____

29) Any behavior, vision, hearing changes or concerns? ☐ No ☐ Yes Describe:_____

30) List preventative medications used (heartworm, flea control): _____

_____

31) Is your pet up-to-date with vaccinations?   ☐ No   ☐ Yes

    List vaccine and dates given:_____

32) Describe your pet's housing environment: _____

33) Does the skin problem itch?   ☐ No   ☐ Yes

VMC #30.3 (Rev. 12/09)   **DERM HISTORY FORM**   **(Please fill out both sides)**

PLACE PATIENT LABEL HERE

Figure 1.1 Dermatology patient history questionnaire. *Source:* Reprinted by permission of the Veterinary Medical Center, University of Minnesota.

34) Does your pet lick?   □ No   □ Yes

If YES, location and frequency_____

35) Does your pet chew?   □ No   □ Yes

If YES, location and frequency_____

36) Does your pet rub?   □ No   □ Yes

If YES, location and frequency_____

37) Does your pet scratch?   □ No   □ Yes

If YES, location and frequency_____

38) Does your pet shake its head frequently?   □ No   □ Yes

39) Is there odor coming from the ears?   □ No   □ Yes

40) Is there discharge coming from the ears?   □ No   □ Yes

41) Does your pet scoot his/her rear end?   □ No   □ Yes

42) Is this problem seasonal?   □ No   □ Yes   □ Unknown

If YES, which seasons?

□ Spring   □ Summer   □ Fall   □ Winter

43) Is this problem year-round?   □ No   □ Yes   □ Unknown

If YES, which season(s) is/are worse?

□ Spring   □ Summer   □ Fall   □ Winter

44) Has you pet been allergy tested?   □ No   □ Yes

If YES, was it a: □ Skin test   □ Blood Test   □ Both skin & blood test   □ Unknown

If YES, has your pet been on allergy shots?   □ No   □ Yes

If YES, response to allergy shots _____

45) Has your pet been on a food trial?   □ No   □ Yes   □ Unknown

If YES, which food?_____

Response to food trial_____

46) Duration of food trial? _____

47) Was any chewable medication (including heartworm) given during food trial?   □ No   □ Yes

48) Number of bowel movements per day?_____

49) Fleas/Lice/Ticks/other parasite problems in the home? _____

50) Flea and Tick control products? (Type/freq) _____

51) How often do you bathe your pet?_____

52) What kind of shampoo and conditioners are used?_____

53) What improves skin condition? _____

54) Percentage time spent indoors?_____%

55) Other pets in the household?   □ No   □ Yes

If YES, include species?_____

56) Exposure to other animals outside of household?   □ No   □ Yes

57) Any other animals in the household affected?   □ No   □ Yes

58) Any humans in the household affected?   □ No   □ Yes

Please list any other questions or concerns_____

_____

_____

_____

_____

VMC #30.3 (Rev. 12/09)   **DERM HISTORY FORM**   **(Please fill out both sides)**

Figure 1.1 (Continued)

which diseases may be more likely to affect them. Examples of important questions to ask the owner of a pet with dermatological signs include: Is the pet itchy? When did they first notice the problem? How has it changed over time? If they have been seen elsewhere for the skin problem, what diagnostic tests have been performed? What medications and treatments have been tried? What has worked for the patient and what hasn't? Is the pet taking any current medications (including over-the-counter products)? Did the medication help to improve the skin lesions and/or reduce the pet's itching? What is the pet's dietary history (including treats)? Is this a seasonal or non-seasonal problem? Are there other pets in the household and if so, are they showing similar signs? Are any humans in the household affected? Good communication and listening skills are essential to obtaining an accurate history.

It is helpful to start at the beginning and get a chronological sequence of events. This can be challenging, as the client may not think that the past information is relevant and may only want to discuss the current issues. Patience and persistence are often required in order to obtain the complete history. And sometimes it is necessary to ask the questions differently in order to get accurate information. For example, you may notice that the dog has alopecia and saliva staining on the paws. You assume the dog has been licking or chewing at his feet. You ask the owner if the dog is itchy (knowing that pruritus can be exhibited by scratching, licking, chewing, or rubbing behavior). The client may only think of scratching as a sign of itching, and will answer "no" to your question. You may then need to ask the client specific questions such as: Have you observed your dog licking, chewing, rubbing, or scratching? If the answer is yes, follow-up questions to ask include: What areas of the body, how often does this occur, and how intense is the licking, chewing, rubbing, and scratching? Each response should be documented in the medical record. You can also ask the client to rate their pet's level of pruritus on a numerical scale of 0–10 (with 0 being none to 10 being constant itching). Providing clients with a visual analog scale (VAS) that includes behavioral descriptions of pruritus can help standardize owner responses (Bergvall 2012, http://www.cliniciansbrief.com/sitesDefault/files/CaninepruritusScale.pdf). The VAS may be more sensitive (Miller et al. 2013) than the numerical scale. This pruritus score can be used to compare the patient's progress at follow-up visits. Pruritus is often the presenting complaint, especially if the pet sleeps in the owner's bedroom and is keeping them awake at night.

Collecting a thorough history can be time consuming, and the veterinary hospital may want to allow additional time for these appointments. Ideally, the person with the most knowledge about the patient should be the person present for the exam. This should be explained to the client when they are scheduling the appointment. A comprehensive history can help the veterinarian develop the most efficient and cost-effective diagnostic and treatment plan for the patient.

Dermatological Procedures

In order to make a diagnosis, the patient history, physical examination findings (see Figure 1.2), and diagnostic tests are used. It is often the veterinary technician's job to perform the diagnostic testing and it is important that the procedure be performed correctly. Keep in mind that a negative test result does not always rule out a disease. The following procedures are often performed on the dermatology patient.

Flea Combing

This technique is used to look for fleas and/or flea dirt (flea feces) if fleas are not found visually on physical exam.

Procedure (Figures 1.3–1.6):

1) Using an ultra-fine flea comb, comb the pet's hair coat thoroughly. You may get lucky and find the adult flea! If not:

a) Place the collected debris on white paper.
b) Wet the debris with water and look for a reddish tinge that indicates dried blood. If positive, this reddish tinge could be from either flea feces or a crust. The next step is to examine the debris microscopically to determine if the debris is flea feces (flea feces are comma shaped).

DERMATOLOGY EXAM
UNIVERSITY OF MINNESOTA
VETERINARY MEDICAL CENTER

Date				Student/Tech	PLACE PATIENT LABEL HERE
Attending Clinician				Diagnostic/Recheck (circle)	
Wt (*Kg/Lbs*)	Temp	Pulse	Resp	Time since last exam	

Progress: Improved Worsened Static

Main Complaint: _____

Problem Started: _____

Progression: _____

_____Other: _____

_____

_____

FeLV: + − unknown   **FIV:** + − unknown

Therapies: (oral / topical)

- Previous _____
  - Response _____
- Current _____

_____

  - Response _____

Pruritus: (circle) Licking Chewing Rubbing Scratching Reporter: _____

Pruritus Visual Analog Scale: _____ Observer: _____

☐ Year-round worse: S SU F W   ☐ Seasonal: S SU F W

Allergy Shots: Previously Currently Never   Response: + − Unknown

Food Trial: Currently Yes No Trial Diet: _____ Response: + − Unknown

Duration: _____ Strict Trial: Yes No # of Bowel movements/day: _____

Diet: (Including treats & snacks) Current_____

Current on HW medication: Yes No Chewable Nonchewable

Environment:_____% time spent indoors _____ outdoors _____ Swims: + −

Amount of contact with: Grass _____ Wool _____ Cement _____ *[none=1, rare=2, some=3, alot=4]*

Exposure to other animals? Dog + − Cats + − Others _____

Others affected? Dog + − Cats + − People + −

Flea Control:

VMC #30.2 (rev. 12/09)   Dermatology Exam

Figure 1.2 Dermatology physical exam form. *Source:* Reprinted by permission of the Veterinary Medical Center, University of Minnesota.

Physical Exam:

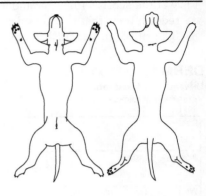

Problem	Rule Out	PLAN Dx	PLAN Rx

Diagnostic Procedures: _____

Cytology: Ear   _____

                Skin _____

Trichogram: _____

Skin scrapings: _____

FNA: _____**Cultures:** Yes _____ No   **Biopsy:**   Yes   No

Clinical Diagnosis _____

Figure 1.2 (Continued)

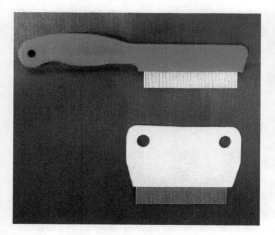

Figure 1.3 Flea combs.

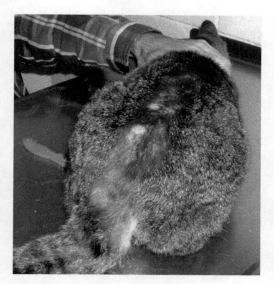

Figure 1.4 Cat with alopecia along dorsal lumbosacral area.

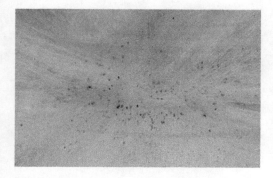

Figure 1.5 Flea excrement, often referred to as "flea dirt."

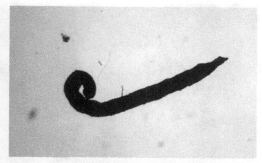

Figure 1.6 Microscopic view of flea feces.

Ear Cytology/Swab

This procedure is used to identify yeast and bacteria. Always swab both ears even if only one ear appears to be affected. Bacterial organisms can be identified morphologically as cocci or rods. *Malassezia pachydermatis* is the most common fungal organism present in ears. The budding yeast usually appears as a peanut or footprint shaped form. Make sure you examine cytology before adding any products into the ears in case a bacterial culture and susceptibility test is indicated.

Procedure when looking for bacteria and yeast (Figures 1.7–1.13):

1) Gently pull up on the ear pinna (see Chapter 4 for an ear diagram) to straighten out the ear canal and insert a cotton-tipped applicator swab into the bottom of vertical ear canal and rotate.
2) Roll the swab onto a labeled microscope slide and heat fix if this is standard for your practice.
3) Stain with Diff-Quik® or new methylene blue.
4) Examine microscopically under an oil immersion lens, 100×. Be sure the microscope is set so the light is up, the condenser is up and open, and the contrast is low. This will allow for the best viewing of yeast and bacteria. These settings should be employed anytime your subjects are cells or infectious agents. (Note: If you are not finding much on the slide, look for epithelial cells with evidence of bacteria and yeast.)

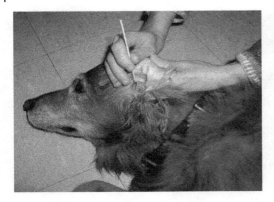

Figure 1.7 Gently pulling up on earflap, insert swab to bottom of vertical ear canal and rotate.

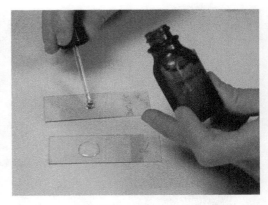

Figure 1.10 Add immersion oil to the stained slide and examine microscopically under an oil immersion lens, 100×.

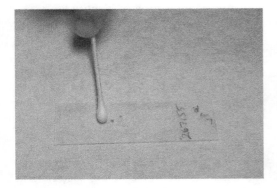

Figure 1.8 Roll swab onto labeled microscope slide.

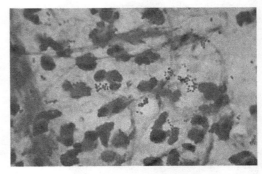

Figure 1.11 Cytologic examination of smear demonstrating cocci bacteria.

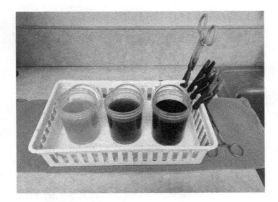

Figure 1.9 Diff-Quik stains. *Source:* Courtesy of Judy K. Lethbridge, CVT, Veterinary Dermatology Center, Maitland, FL.

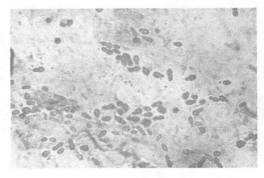

Figure 1.12 Cytologic examination of smear demonstrating *Malassezia* yeast.

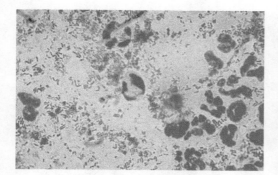

Figure 1.13 Cytologic examination of smear demonstrating rod bacteria.

Samples collected for bacterial culture should follow step 1 above, utilizing sterile swabs and aseptic technique.

Procedure when looking for *Otodectes/ Demodex/Sarcoptes* mites and/or eggs (Figures 1.14–1.17):

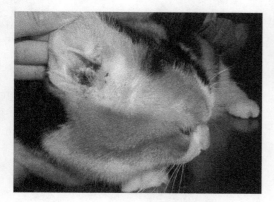

Figure 1.14 Cat with classic coffee ground appearance of discharge due to infestation of ear mites. Excoriations likely from scratching are also noted on the pinna.

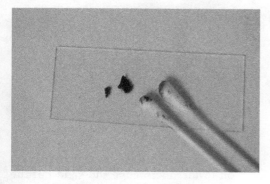

Figure 1.15 Close up of ear debris collected by swab.

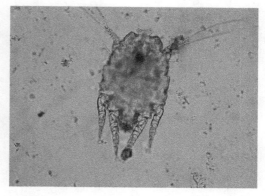

Figure 1.16 Adult *Otodectes* mite.

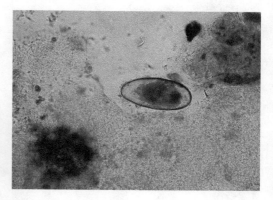

Figure 1.17 *Otodectes* egg.

1) Apply a few drops of mineral oil into the ears and onto a microscope slide.
2) Moisten a cotton swab with mineral oil.
3) Insert the swab into the ear canal and collect debris.
4) Place the collected material in the mineral oil on the microscope slide.
5) Apply a coverslip (if desired) and examine microscopically under 4× or 10×. For the best visualization of mites, set the microscope so the light is low, the condenser is down and closed, and the contrast is increased. These settings should be employed anytime your subjects are parasites.

Skin Cytology

Skin cytology is an underused diagnostic test that is easy to perform, relatively quick and inexpensive, and can provide a wealth of information. The following techniques can be used.

Tape Prep (Especially Useful for Finding Yeast on the Skin)
Procedure (Figures 1.18–1.23):

1) Use clear sticky tape.
2) Firmly press the sticky side onto the skin area to be sampled and vigorously rub the back of the tape. Use one of the staining method options below:

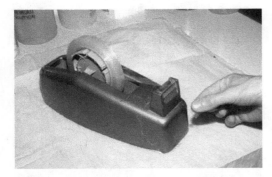

Figure 1.18 Clear, one-sided sticky tape.

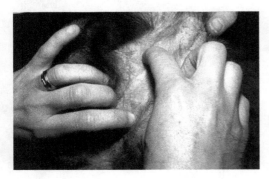

Figure 1.19 Press sticky side onto skin area to be sampled and vigorously rub back of tape.

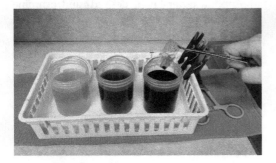

Figure 1.20 Stain tape with a third (purple) stain of Diff-Quik. *Source:* Courtesy of Judy K. Lethbridge, CVT, Veterinary Dermatology Center, Maitland, FL.

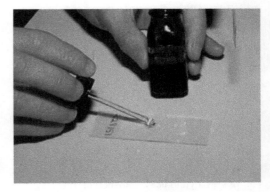

Figure 1.21 Apply immersion oil to microscope slide.

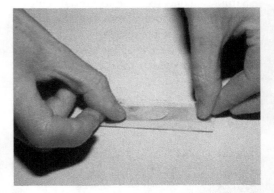

Figure 1.22 Put stained tape sticky side down.

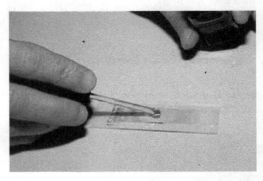

Figure 1.23 Apply immersion oil on top of tape and examine microscopically under an oil immersion lens, 100×.

3a) Stain the tape with a third (purple) stain of Diff-Quik. Rinse the tape and gently blot dry on a paper towel. Apply immersion oil to the microscope slide and put the tape sticky side down.

3b) Apply a drop of new methylene blue stain to the slide and put the tape sticky side down.

4) Apply immersion oil on top of the tape and examine under an oil immersion lens, 100×. (Note: You may want to scan the slide on low power to find areas of interest before applying immersion oil.)

Alternate methods:

1) A dry, dull scalpel blade or scraping spatula can also be used to gently scrape oily or moist skin surfaces to obtain a sample. Collected material is placed on a slide, heat fixed (if standard for your practice), and stained with Diff-Quik (Figures 1.24–1.26).

2) Cotton-tipped applicator swabs can be used to collect samples from oily or

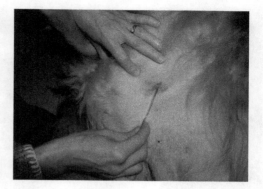

Figure 1.26 A dry spatula is used to gently scrape the skin surface to collect skin cytology.

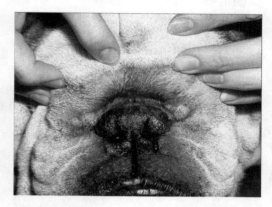

Figure 1.27 Oily or moist skin surfaces that may be difficult to access to collect cytology include interdigital areas and facial folds.

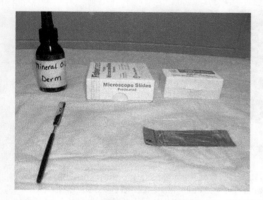

Figure 1.24 Alternatives to tape prep technique include using a dry scalpel blade or spatula to collect the sample.

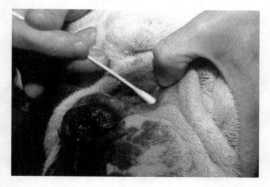

Figure 1.28 Cotton swab used to collect sample from the nasal fold of an English bulldog.

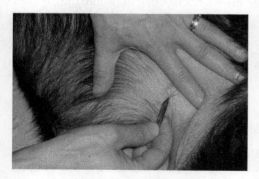

Figure 1.25 A dry #10 scalpel blade is used to carefully scrape the skin surface to collect skin cytology.

moist skin surfaces that are difficult to access, such as interdigital areas, facial folds, and tail folds (Figures 1.27 and 1.28).

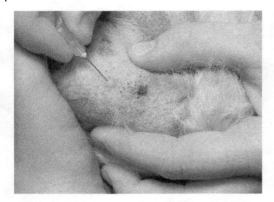

Figure 1.29 Gently break open a pustule with a 25 gauge needle.

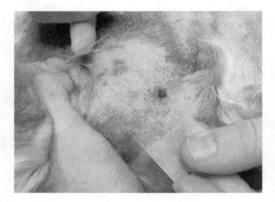

Figure 1.30 Press a microscope slide onto the ruptured pustule to collect a sample.

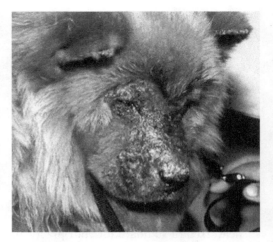

Figure 1.31 Chow Chow with facial crusts. Gently lift up a crust and press a microscope slide onto exposed skin, or press the undersurface of the crust onto the slide.

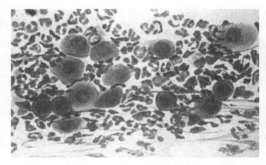

Figure 1.32 Cytologic examination showing acantholytic cells (large round cells) suggestive of the autoimmune disease pemphigus.

Sampling a Pustule

Procedure (Figures 1.29 and 1.30):

1) Gently break open a pustule with a 25 gauge needle.
2) Press a microscope slide onto the ruptured pustule.
3) Allow the sample to air dry or heat fix.
4) Stain with Diff-Quik.
5) Examine under an oil immersion lens, 100×.

Samples collected for bacterial culture follow step 1 above, utilizing sterile swabs and aseptic technique.

Sampling a Crust

Procedure (Figures 1.31 and 1.32):

1) Gently lift up the crust.
2) Press a microscope slide onto the exposed skin or press the undersurface of the crust onto the slide.
3) Allow the sample to air dry or heat fix.
4) Stain with Diff-Quik.
5) Examine under an oil immersion lens, 100×.

Skin Scraping

Different techniques are used depending on which mite you are searching for. A good history will help determine which mites you should be suspicious of.

Sarcoptes scabiei and *Notoedres cati* (Feline Scabies)

Multiple superficial scrapings are needed; you may still only find sarcoptic mites approximately 20% of the time (Miller et al. 2013).

Procedure (Figures 1.33–1.37):

1) Put mineral oil on a microscope slide.
2) Either dip a #10 scalpel blade or a scraping spatula into oil or apply oil directly to the skin site. (Note: Prior to scraping, dull the scalpel blade to prevent accidentally cutting the patient.)
3) Pick an area that is crusty but not too excoriated or inflamed to scrape. Scrape a broad area about the size of your palm superficially.

(a)

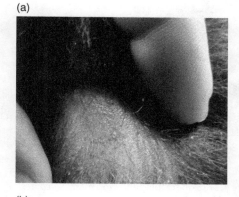

(b)

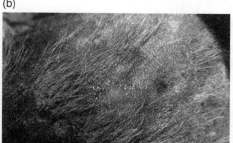

Figure 1.35 (a) and (b) Scrape deep enough to get capillary oozing. Remember that multiple scrapings are needed. *Source:* Courtesy of Judy K. Lethbridge, CVT, Veterinary Dermatology Center, Maitland, FL.

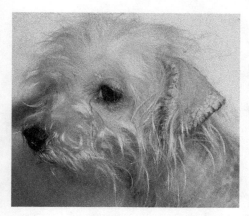

Figure 1.33 Dog with sarcoptic mange. Skin lesions include erythema, alopecia, scaling, crusts, and ear margin fissures.

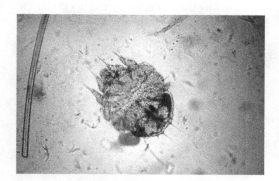

Figure 1.36 Skin scraping showing an adult *Sarcoptes* mite.

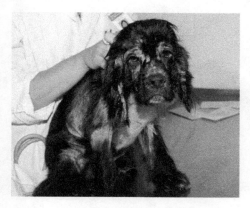

Figure 1.34 Ten-month Cocker Spaniel with sarcoptic mange. Patient was being treated for allergies after initial skin scrapings were negative.

4) Put samples on labeled slides and apply a coverslip.
5) Examine the samples thoroughly under the microscope at 10× or 20×.

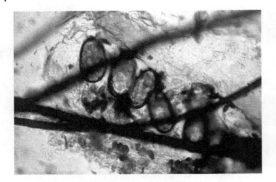

Figure 1.37 Skin scraping showing many *Sarcoptes* eggs and fecal pellets.

Demodex canis, Demodex cati, Demodex injai

Procedure (Figures 1.38–1.41):

1) Choose three to four sites to sample.
2) Put mineral oil on a microscope slide.
3) Either dip a dull #10 scalpel blade or scraping spatula in oil or apply oil directly to the skin site.
4) Squeeze the skin (to help extrude mites from the hair follicle).
5) Scrape deeply enough to get capillary oozing (blood should be evident on the slide).
6) Put samples on labeled slides and apply a coverslip.
7) Examine the samples thoroughly under the microscope at 10× or 20×. (Note: Lowering

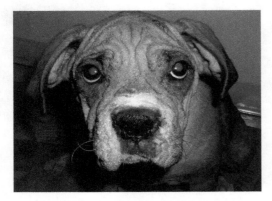

Figure 1.38 Boxer puppy with generalized demodicosis. Skin lesions include alopecia, erythema, papules, pustules, and hyperpigmentation.

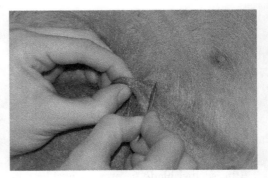

Figure 1.39 Scraping deep enough to get capillary oozing and squeezing the skin will help extrude mites from the hair follicle. *Source:* Dr. Sheila Torres, courtesy of the University of Minnesota, College of Veterinary Medicine.

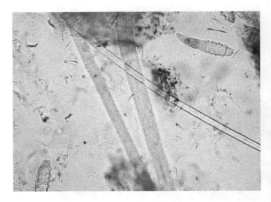

Figure 1.40 Skin scraping showing adult *Demodex* mites (four pairs of legs).

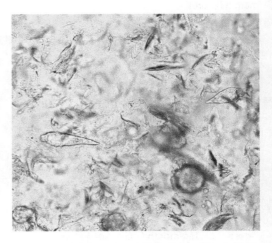

Figure 1.41 Skin scraping showing a larval stage (three pairs of legs) and an egg (fusiform shape) of *Demodex*.

Box 1.1 Example of Documenting Skin Scraping Results of the Demodex Mite Stages

Location: _____
    Adults (alive):_____
    Adults (dead):_____
    Nymphs: _____
    Larvae: _____
    Eggs: _____

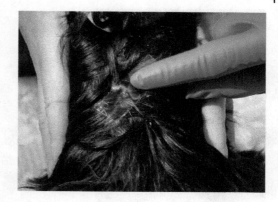

Figure 1.43 Spread the hair and use clear sticky tape to press onto the skin and scale. *Source:* Courtesy of Judy K. Lethbridge, CVT, Veterinary Dermatology Center, Maitland, FL.

the microscope condenser to increase contrast will help with mite visualization.)

8) Count mites or at least record stages of mites found from each area scraped and document in the medical record (see Box 1.1). This information will be used to monitor the treatment response.

Cheyletiella spp., Demodex cornei, Demodex gatoi, Lynxacarus radovsky, Lice (Linognathus setosus, Trichodectes canis, Felicola subrostratus, etc.)

Procedure (Figures 1.42 and 1.43):

1) Multiple samples are needed, and may still be difficult to find.
2) Put mineral oil on a microscope slide and use one or all of the following methods:
   a) Dip a dull #10 blade or scraping spatula in oil and do broad superficial skin scraping.
   b) Use clear tape, press onto the skin and scale (usually the dorsal area for *cheyletiella*).
   c) Flea combing to collect hair, scale, and debris.
3) Put samples on labeled slides and apply a coverslip.
4) Examine the samples thoroughly under the microscope at 10× or 20×.

Fecal Flotation

This technique can be used to look for *Cheyletiella spp.* and *D. gatoi* (feline) if skin scrapings are negative. These mites live superficially in the skin and can be ingested by the pruritic pet when it grooms itself (Figures 1.44–1.46).

Trichography

A trichogram can be used to look for fungal arthrospores in cases of suspected dermatophytosis; to determine the growth phase of the hair; to look for lice eggs, *cheyletiella* eggs, or *demodex* mites adhered to the hair; or to determine if the tips of the hairs are broken off.

Procedure (Figures 1.47–1.50):

1) Pluck suspicious hairs with a forceps in the direction of the hair growth.
2) Place hairs in mineral oil on a microscope slide and apply a coverslip.
3) Scan microscopically under low power and increase magnification as needed.

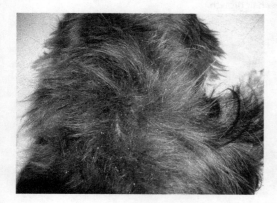

Figure 1.42 Puppy with cheyletiellosis. Skin lesions include scaling over dorsum.

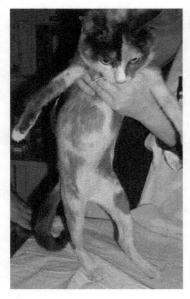

Figure 1.44 If skin scrapings are negative, fecal flotation may be used to look for *Cheyletiella spp.* and *Demodex gatoi* (feline). These mites live superficially in the skin and can be ingested by the pruritic cat. Alopecic feline patient with *D. gatoi.*

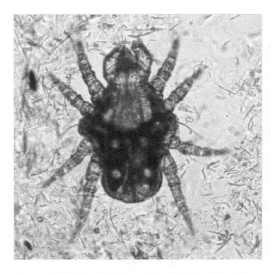

Figure 1.46 *Cheyletiella spp. Source:* Courtesy of Dr. Karen Moriello, Clinical Professor of Dermatology, School of Veterinary Medicine, University of Wisconsin-Madison.

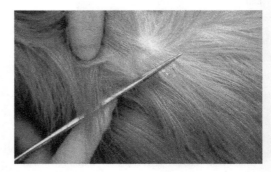

Figure 1.47 To perform a trichogram, pluck suspicious hairs with a forceps in the direction of the hair growth.

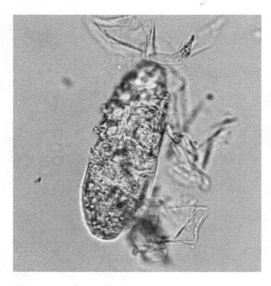

Figure 1.45 *Demodex gatoi.*

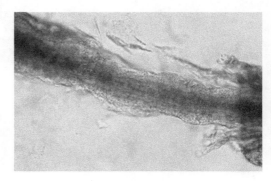

Figure 1.48 Trichogram showing an infected hair with arthrospores.

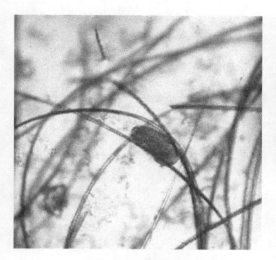

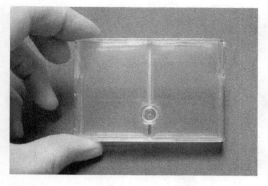

Figure 1.51 Example of a flat fungal culture bi-plate – dermatophyte test medium (amber color) and Sabouraud's dextrose agar.

Figure 1.49 Trichogram showing a *Cheyletiella* mite egg.

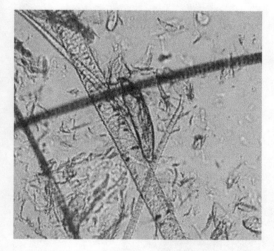

Figure 1.50 Trichogram showing a *Demodex* mite adhered to the hair.

Dermatophyte Culture

A dermatophyte culture is often necessary to diagnose dermatophytosis. Dermatophyte test medium (DTM) is frequently used in private practice (Figure 1.51). This medium contains a phenol red indicator that may turn the medium red. This color change can occur with both dermatophytes and saprophytes (contaminants). Therefore, it is important to check these cultures daily or every other day to observe how soon color change and colony growth occur. Dermatophytes typically turn the media red much earlier than saprophytes, often within 7–10 days. The color change needs to occur prior to or in conjunction with colony growth to be significant.

Procedure:

1) Pluck suspicious hairs (broken or mis-shapen hairs; hairs associated with scale, crust, or inflammation; or hairs with positive fluorescence under a Wood's lamp) that are close to the edge of the lesion, or use the Mackenzie brush technique to collect hairs from clinically normal patients.
2) Gently press collected hairs onto DTM culture.
3) Incubate DTM in a darkened area at room temperature, ideally around 30° centi-grade and 30% humidity (Miller et al. 2013).
4) DTM culture should be aerobic.
5) Keep culture for a minimum of three to four weeks before calling negative. (Note: Patients already on treatment for derma-tophytosis may take longer to show growth on culture.)
6) Perform tape prep to identify a colony microscopically. (Note: If you have a sus-picious colony that is in danger of being overgrown by a saprophyte, you can inoc-ulate the suspicious colony onto a new DTM plate.)

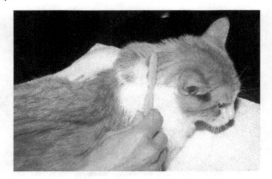

Figure 1.52 Mackenzie Brush Technique-brushing cat with toothbrush.

Mackenzie Brush Technique

This technique is particularly useful for asymptomatic patients (including patients on treatment whose clinical signs have resolved).

Procedure (Figure 1.52):

1) Remove a new, unopened toothbrush from its package and brush the entire patient head to toe.
2) Pay special attention to collecting hair from face and ears.
3) Press the toothbrush with hairs gently onto DTM.
   a) You may need to remove hairs from the toothbrush with a needle, scalpel blade, or forceps.
   b) For ease of placing the hair sample onto DTM, it is preferred to use flat culture plates for this technique.

Tape Prep Procedure

A method used to identify colony growth on DTM.

Procedure (Figures 1.53–1.56):

1) Place a drop of lactophenol cotton blue or new methylene blue stain on a microscope slide.
2) Use clear, one-sided sticky tape.
3) Grab the tape with forceps and lightly press onto the colony.
4) Place the tape, sticky side down, on the slide and apply a coverslip.
5) For ease of collection, it is preferable to use flat culture plates for this procedure.
6) Examine under 10× and then 40× to identify macroconidia.

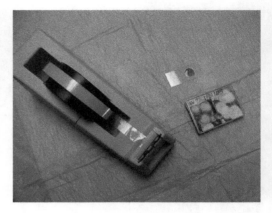

Figure 1.53 Supplies (sticky tape, stain, and dermatophyte test medium) for tape prep of colony growth.

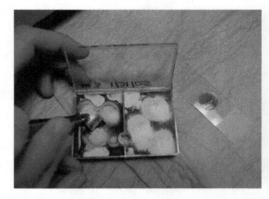

Figure 1.54 Lightly press one-sided sticky tape onto suspicious colony.

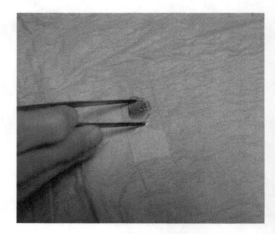

Figure 1.55 Press collected material on tape into stain on microscope slide.

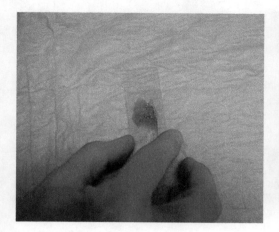

Figure 1.56 Apply coverslip.

Skin Punch Biopsy

Multiple biopsies should be taken and ideally sent to a dermatohistopathologist. Including the patient signalment, complete history, physical exam findings including type and location of skin lesions, list of differential diagnoses, and pictures (if possible) along with the submitted samples will help to obtain the correct diagnosis. Skin biopsies can often be obtained with local anesthesia only. However, some inflamed or deep lesions (e.g. panniculitis) do not block well with local anesthetic, so sedation or general anesthesia may be necessary as determined by the veterinarian.

Procedure (Figures 1.57–1.64):

1) The veterinarian indicates sites to be biopsied. Only affected skin should be

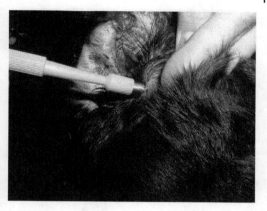

Figure 1.58 Gently press the biopsy punch over the site and begin to rotate the punch in one direction to collect the sample.

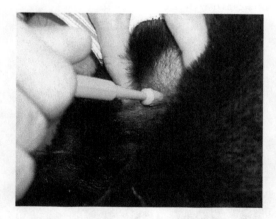

Figure 1.59 Continue rotating until you feel the punch go through the skin (depending on the thickness of the skin in the area you are sampling, the entire hub of the punch may be embedded).

(a)

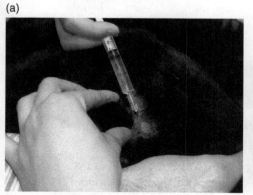

(b)

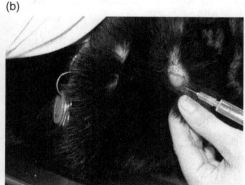

Figure 1.57 (a and b) Injecting lidocaine subcutaneously under each biopsy site.

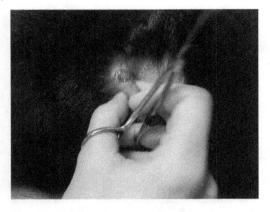

Figure 1.60 When deep enough, remove the punch and grab the sample gently with fingers. If you cannot use your fingers, then try gently stabbing the sample with a 25 gauge needle to lift the skin (using a forceps may crush the tissue).

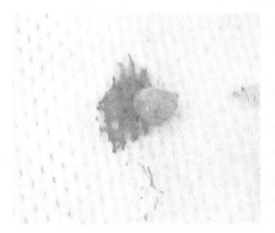

Figure 1.62 Dry the biopsy skin sample gently with gauze.

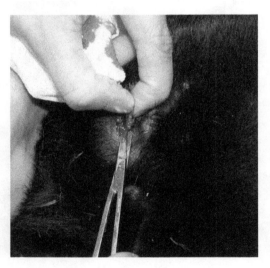

Figure 1.61 Gently lift the sample and cut as deeply as possible with an iris scissor.

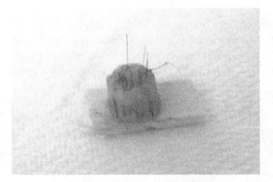

Figure 1.63 Place the sample hair side up on a piece of tongue depressor.

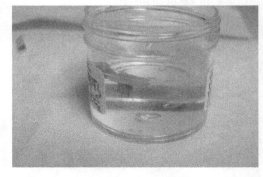

Figure 1.64 Put the sample hair side down in a jar of 10% buffered formalin.

included. If normal skin is needed to be sent to the dermatohistopathologist, this sample should be marked as such and submitted in a separate container.

2) Inject 0.5–1.0 ml of lidocaine subcutaneously under each site (intradermal injection can cause artifacts in the sample).

  a) Do not exceed 1 ml per 5 kg body weight to prevent cardiac arrhythmias (Mueller 2004).

3) Wait a few minutes for lidocaine to take effect before beginning.

4) **Do not** disturb the skin in any way prior to taking the biopsy. This includes shaving and scrubbing, as doing so can remove crusts which may be needed to make a diagnosis.

(Note: If the biopsy site is not alopecic, a scissors can be used to gently trim away excess hair to allow the biopsy punch to have closer contact with the skin.)

5) Usually a 4, 6, or 8 mm punch is used (6 or 8 mm preferred unless obtaining a sample from areas such as nasal planum or footpad). Tissue will shrink once placed in formalin.

6) Place the punch over the center of the lesion and rotate the punch in one direction to collect a sample.

7) When deep enough, remove the punch and grasp the sample gently with fingers (to avoid pinching or crushing of skin). If using forceps, gently grasp subcutaneous tissue rather than skin.

8) Gently lift up the sample and cut as deeply as possible with iris scissors.

9) Apply pressure with a gauze pad to the biopsy site as needed for hemostasis, then close with suture material.

10) Gently blot the underside of the biopsy sample on dry gauze.

11) Place the sample hair side up on a piece of tongue depressor (this allows the tissue orientation to be preserved for sample preparation at the histopathology lab).

12) Put the sample hair side down in a jar of 10% buffered formalin.

Skin biopsies may also be used to collect samples for aerobic and anaerobic bacterial and fungal cultures. For this procedure, the skin site is disinfected and samples collected aseptically and placed into the appropriate transport media. The laboratory should be contacted for specific instructions and materials for collection.

Client Education and Client Compliance

Patients with dermatological diseases can require a lot of at-home care. Owners who have a good understanding of their pet's disease are more likely to comply with therapeutic recommendations. For example, if the veterinarian prescribes a medicated antibacterial or antifungal shampoo to be used twice weekly, and the shampoo should have a 10–15 minute contact time, the technician should explain how this treatment will benefit the patient. If owners understand the process, they will be more likely to use the medicated shampoo as prescribed. This is how the author explains the allergic process to the owner: "When your dog eats or absorbs (either through the skin or inhalation) something it is allergic to, the skin becomes inflamed (you may notice pink or red skin). The skin may also become greasy and this inflammation and greasiness provide a great environment for bacteria and yeast. Because this inflamed skin is no longer a good barrier, the microorganisms that normally live on the skin surface are able to proliferate and cause an infection. The infection increases the level of itchiness. Using this medicated shampoo will decrease the number of microorganisms on the skin surface and hopefully will decrease the itching." Make sure the owner is aware that the shampoo is working while the pet is lathered up, so the veterinarian's recommended contact time is important.

Emphasize to the client the expectations of treatment. Does their pet have a disease that cannot be cured but only controlled? If curable, will the condition take a long time to reach a cure, and will the treatment involve a substantial time commitment and/or financial commitment from the owner? If the disease is only controllable, make sure clients understand that it may take some trial and error to establish the ideal treatment plan for each individual patient. Let them know that you will work together with them as a team to find out what treatment plan will work the best to make their pet the most comfortable.

Recheck appointments are critical to the successful management of each patient. Always recheck ear and skin infection patients prior to discontinuing antimicrobial therapy. The rule of thumb is to continue treatment of superficial infections for one to two weeks past clinical resolution of signs

(Koch et al. 2012; Miller et al. 2013). Deep skin infections will require longer treatment, a minimum of 4 weeks and often up to 12 weeks, and therapy should be continued for 2 weeks past clinical resolution of signs (Koch et al. 2012; Miller et al. 2013). Patients with parasitic skin diseases (especially demodicosis) as well as patients with dermatophytosis often look clinically normal before the condition is actually cured. Stopping treatment too soon will likely result in a relapse. Clients need to understand the importance of these rechecks so that they keep their appointments.

Some ectoparasite infestations can be prevented. It is much easier and less expensive to prevent ectoparasite infestations rather than paying to treat the primary condition along with all its secondary complications. Especially in regions that can support flea survival year round, dogs and cats with flea allergy dermatitis should always be on flea prevention. In addition, since many diseases such as tapeworms, babesiosis, anaplasmosis, and ehrlichiosis can be transmitted to our pets by fleas and ticks, ectoparasite control is an important aspect of maintaining overall patient health. It is likely the veterinary technician will be involved in educating clients and assisting them in choosing a preventative product for their pet. Improving clients' knowledge about fleas and setting realistic owner expectations is a very important factor in achieving success with flea control (Dryden 2009). Veterinary technicians who educate the client and set realistic expectations can be a valuable asset to the veterinary practice.

Many skin conditions have underlying causes, which will be important to investigate if the problem continues to recur. Mentioning this to the client and letting them know that further diagnostic tests or a referral to a dermatologist might be indicated in the future may help prevent a client from becoming frustrated and dissatisfied with the veterinary care their pet received at your practice.

Helpful Hints to Improve Client Compliance

Capsules and Tablets

- For oral administration with capsules directly into the back of the mouth, wetting the capsule with water will help it slide down easier (rather than sticking to your finger).
- When possible, giving clients the choice of treating their pet with once- or twice-daily antibiotic medications and explaining the cost difference may help improve compliance.
- Often, oral medications are hidden in food, which can be a challenge when the patient is on a food trial. If a canned version of the prescription food trial diet is not available, some options are canned pumpkin, baked potato, oatmeal, and cooked sweet potato. Allergy formula pill pockets may also be an option.

Injections

For patients who dislike receiving their immunotherapy injections:

- Rotate rooms that the injection is administered in.
- Place pet on a table or a slippery surface like a washer/dryer to give the injection (ensuring the patient is safe from falling or jumping off).
- Use positive reinforcement – giving treats during and after the injection. (Note: Putting canned food onto the floor, table, or a plate for them to lick while receiving an injection can be a good distraction in a patient that is not food aggressive.)
- After drawing the allergen dose into the syringe, warm the syringe to room temperature prior to injection.
- Practice pinching up skin and then reward the pet for holding still.
- Practice getting the syringe out and with the cap on pretend to give an injection.
- Remind the owner to remain calm and relaxed, as pets can sense the owner's nervousness.

- Offer to have the veterinary technician administer injections at no charge or for a nominal fee.

Bathing

- Ensure the floor of the bathtub or shower is not slippery by using rubber bath mats.
- Use lukewarm water – inflamed skin is warm and cooler water will be soothing.
- If the patient is dirty, have the client bathe the pet first with a mild shampoo to remove dirt, then use a medicated shampoo.
- If medicated shampoo is thick, dilute with water in a squeeze bottle; this will provide a more even lather of shampoo throughout the hair coat.
- Avoid applying a large amount of shampoo to the dorsal midline to spread from there. Instead, apply a small amount of the shampoo onto hands and then massage into various locations to get an even application to the pet's haircoat.
- Have the client start lathering the most affected area of skin first, then lather up the rest of the body and begin timing the recommended amount of contact time.
- Gently massage shampoo into the skin. Avoid vigorous scrubbing to prevent irritation of already inflamed skin.
- Read a book out loud while waiting to rinse the pet (this may calm the dog to sit still in the tub).
- Use positive rewards (such as feeding treats) while the dog is in the tub.
- If bathing outside, play with the dog or take them for a walk while they are lathered up.
- **Always** rinse thoroughly – when the client thinks they have removed all the shampoo, rinse one more time just to be sure!
- Offer therapeutic bathing services in your hospital.
- Refer client to a self-service dog wash or groomer.

Ear Cleaning

- Demonstrate the proper ear cleaning technique during the appointment (after demonstrating one ear, have the client clean the other ear while you observe).
- Cover the patient with a towel when flushing and massaging ears (keeping the pet clean may increase compliance).
- Grab the ear flap along with the collar when filling the canal to stabilize the patient's head.
- Fill both ears at once to prevent head tilting and then massage.
- For pets that don't tolerate filling the ear canal with solution, have the client saturate a cotton ball with ear cleaner and place into the ear canal, then squeeze the cotton ball to get the cleaner in.
- Some pets may tolerate lying on their side rather than being in a sitting or standing position.
- Warm the ear cleaner solution prior to applying in the ears.
- Use hypoallergenic baby wipes or antimicrobial wipes to clean the ear flap.

Handouts

Handouts are a great way to reinforce what has been explained to the client in the exam room.

- Create handouts for the different diseases and then include the patient's specific recommendations on the back.
- Give clients the handouts to read while you are looking at cytology and skin scrapings, and then answer any questions they have when you come back in the room.
- Having handout templates on the computer that can be customized for each patient's discharge instructions is very efficient.

Recheck Appointment Options

- Schedule the recheck appointment at the end of the initial exam, and give the client a reminder card with the appointment date and time.
- Call the client one to two days after the exam to see how the pet is doing and then schedule the appointment.
- Create a recall list and callback reminders to schedule the recheck.

- Mail out reminder cards when the patient is due and/or after the client has scheduled the recheck appointment. Email or text messages may be preferred by some clients.
- Call the client two days prior to the appointment for confirmation. Sometimes the client may want to cancel their appointment because the pet is better. This is another opportunity for the veterinary technician to educate the client. For example, in the case of a skin or ear infection, the intent was that the patient would respond favorably to treatment; however, the purpose of the recheck is for the veterinarian to repeat cytology and assess how much longer the treatment needs to be continued. If you convince the client to come for the recheck, but the client needs to reschedule to a later date, the patient should receive additional medication to last until the next appointment.

Phone Calls

- Make follow-up phone calls midway through a diet trial.
- Check in with the client when their pet is on a decreasing dose of steroids.
- Give reminders when the patient is due for lab work (especially for patients on long-term corticosteroid or cyclosporine therapy).
- Patient updates: Ensure clients are following discharge instructions correctly. Bring any problems or concerns to the veterinarian's attention if the patient is not doing well.

Conclusion

As a veterinary technician you play a vital role in the management of dermatology patients. Obtaining an accurate history and performing diagnostic procedures correctly are extremely important. Providing thorough client education about the diagnosis and therapeutic recommendations made by the veterinarian is crucial to ensuring client compliance. These fundamental elements are essential for the successful management of the dermatology patient.

References

Bergvall, K. (2012). History, examination and initial evaluation. In: *BSAVA Manual of Canine and Feline Dermatology*, 3e (eds. Jackson H.A and Marsella R.), 16–18. Gloucester: British Small Animal Veterinary Association.

Dryden, M. (2009). Current Challenges in Flea Control. *24th Proceedings of the North American Veterinary Dermatology Forum*. Harrisburg, PA: NAVDF.

Koch, S.N., Torres, S.M.F., and Plumb, D.C. (2012). *Canine and Feline Dermatology Drug Handbook*, 1e. Ames, IA: Wiley Blackwell.

Miller, W.H., Griffin, C.E., and Campbell, K.L. (2013). *Muller and Kirk's Small Animal Dermatology*, 7e. St. Louis, Missouri: Elsevier.

Mueller, R.S. (2004). *Manual for the Small Animal Practice Dermatology Made Easy*. Babenhausen: Teton NM & BE VetVerlag.

Nationwide (2018). Most common medical conditions that prompt veterinary visits. https://press8.petinsurance.com/articles/2018/march/most-common-medical-conditions-that-prompt-veterinary-visits (accessed May 2019).

Section II

Skin and Ear Diseases

2

Bacterial Infections

Dawn Logas and Christie Yamazaki Delan

Introduction

Pyodermas are usually classified by the skin layers that are involved. Surface pyodermas affect mainly the stratum corneum, the outermost layer of the epidermis. Superficial pyodermas affect the entire epidermis and the hair follicles. Deep pyodermas also involve the dermis and occasionally the subcutis (Noli and Morris 2012).

Since this chapter is about common bacterial infections seen in practice, we will limit our discussion to infections caused by Staphylococcal bacteria, primarily *Staphylococcus pseudintermedius*, the *Staphylococcus* species found most commonly on the dog. *Staphylococcus schlieferi* and *Staphylococcus aureus* can also cause canine and feline pyodermas, but are much less common. Detailed information about other bacterial skin infections can be found in references listed in the recommended reading section at the end of this chapter. Canine pyodermas will be discussed in more depth than feline pyodermas, since they are seen much more often in clinical practice.

make up the host epidermal microbiome, whose role in skin function and development is still not completely understood. Under normal circumstances these bacteria are kept in check by the host epidermal barrier and the skin's immune system. The presence of another dermatological disease such as allergic dermatitis, endocrinopathy, autoimmune disease, or parasitic infestation can compromise the epidermal barrier and the skin immune system function. This allows these resident bacteria to multiply and become pathogenic, causing the skin disease commonly referred to as pyoderma. For this reason, these infections are considered a secondary problem. Therefore, diagnosis and control of the underlying disease is essential in the management and prevention of these bacterial infections. Client education is consequently extremely important so the owner understands that not only the active infection must be controlled, but the underlying condition as well.

Pathogenesis

Dogs and cats, like all other mammals, have a variety of bacteria that normally inhabit their skin surface. These bacteria

Surface Pyodermas

Surface pyodermas include pyotraumatic moist dermatitis (hot spots) and intertrigo (skin fold dermatitis).

Small Animal Dermatology for Technicians and Nurses, First Edition. Edited by Kim Horne, Marcia Schwassmann and Dawn Logas.

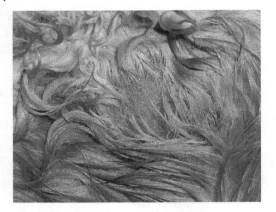

Figure 2.1 Dog with pyotraumatic moist dermatitis on the lateral thigh; note erythema and moist exudate. *Source:* Courtesy of Wayne Rosenkrantz DVM, DACVD, Animal Dermatology Clinic, Tustin, CA.

Clinical Features

Pyotraumatic moist dermatitis (Figure 2.1) is caused, as the name suggests, by self-trauma, usually licking. Therefore, areas of moist dermatitis found in places where the dog cannot lick such as under the ear are not true hot spots and will be discussed later in this chapter. Hot spots are usually extremely pruritic and can come up within a few hours. They are frequently associated with flea bite allergy, so are commonly found on the caudal half of the body. They consist of an erythematous, moist, partially to completely alopecic, exudative area of skin that is pruritic and sometimes painful to the touch.

Intertrigo can develop in any dog with skin folds. This condition is common in brachycephalic breeds such as pugs and English bulldogs, but can also be seen in obese dogs of any breed. The lesions can be found anywhere there are skin folds. Some of the more commonly affected areas are the face, ventral neck, axillae, intermammary space, perivulvar fold, and tail fold (Figures 2.2–2.4). The lesions usually consist of an area of swollen, erythematous skin that is odiferous and moist. In severe cases the skin may be eroded or ulcerated and painful. Pruritus varies from absent to severe.

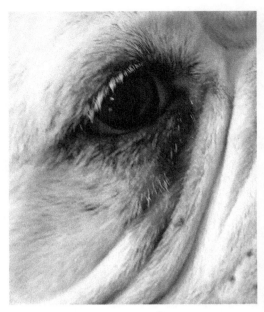

Figure 2.2 Intertrigo of facial fold area. *Source:* Courtesy of Amy Weller, Dermatology Clinic for Animals, Tacoma, WA.

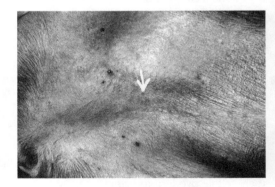

Figure 2.3 Dog with intertrigo of umbilical fold (white arrow). *Source:* Courtesy of Wayne Rosenkrantz DVM, DACVD, Animal Dermatology Clinic, Tustin, CA.

Surface pyodermas are also seen in areas of chronic dermatitis where the skin has thickened and lichenified, forming small folds and crevices (Figure 2.5). These areas can also be fairly odiferous with a great deal of exudate. They are usually pruritic.

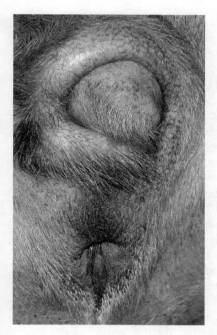

Figure 2.4 Dog with intertrigo of tail fold; note the swollen appearance and hyperpigmentation.

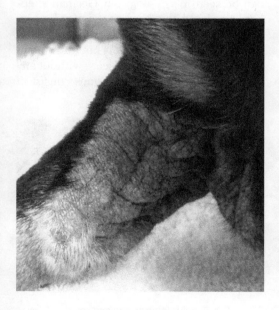

Figure 2.5 Dog with chronic dermatitis showing alopecia, lichenification, and hyperpigmentation in the axilla. *Source:* Courtesy of Amy Weller, Dermatology Clinic for Animals, Tacoma, WA.

Diagnostic Tests

Pyotraumatic dermatitis and intertrigo usually present with a classic history and clinical appearance, so are typically diagnosed on physical examination. Cytology should be done to look for the presence of inflammatory cells, bacteria, and yeast. With pyotraumatic moist dermatitis, you would expect to find bacteria on your cytology. Intertrigo can be associated with both bacteria and yeast overgrowths. By identifying the bacteria as cocci (usually *Staphylococcus sp.*) or rods (*Pseudomonas, Proteus, or Escherichia coli*), the cytology will help determine which topical therapies will be best to use.

It is also important to look for the underlying cause of the surface bacterial infection. Pyotraumatic dermatitis can be associated with poor hygiene, ectoparasitic infestations, and allergic dermatitis. Intertrigo is often simply the result of breed-specific anatomy, but can be complicated by allergic dermatitis or other diseases that affect the skin's barrier function and immune system function. The patient's history and other clinical signs will determine what additional diagnostic testing the veterinarian will recommend.

Treatment

Treatment for surface pyodermas usually consists of topical therapy. The use of an antimicrobial shampoo is recommended. The antimicrobials may be delivered in a mousse, spray, or wipe-on preparation instead of or in addition to the shampoo. Many times a topical antibacterial/steroid preparation is needed to clear up the active infection and decrease the pruritus. Areas of pyotraumatic dermatitis should be clipped so they can be appropriately cleaned and medicated. The patient may need to be sedated for clipping if the hot spot is pruritic and painful. If the hot spot is secondary to flea exposure, it is very important to get the patient on a good flea control program to prevent the hot spot from recurring. The patient may also need to wear an Elizabethan collar for several days until the pruritus has abated. This will minimize additional self-trauma.

Systemic antibiotics are usually not needed and are not recommended for most surface infections unless they are severely ulcerated and painful. A short course of an oral anti-inflammatory agent such as prednisone may be required for severely pruritic hot spots.

Superficial Pyodermas

Superficial pyodermas include impetigo, folliculitis, and mucocutaneous pyoderma.

Clinical Features

Impetigo (Figure 2.6) presents as pustules that are not centered on hair follicles. This disorder is mainly seen on the ventral abdomen and inguinal area of young dogs (less than one year of age). Impetigo can occur spontaneously or can be associated with

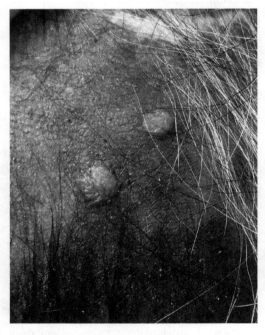

Figure 2.6 Impetigo; note the large, non-follicular pustules. *Source:* Courtesy of Wayne Rosenkrantz DVM, DACVD, Animal Dermatology Clinic, Tustin, California.

endoparasitism or poor hygiene. The condition is usually not pruritic and is easily cleared with topical antibacterial therapy.

Bacterial folliculitis can be seen in any age, sex, and breed of dog. Clients may complain of increased odor that returns quickly, even after bathing. Increased shedding may also be reported. The lesions of bacterial folliculitis are normally found on the trunk and usually spare the head, ears, and forelimbs. The lesions consist of papules, pustules, epidermal collarettes, crusts, and patchy alopecia (Figures 2.7–2.9). The skin may be erythematous in the active stages, but there may also be areas of post-inflammatory hyper- or hypo-pigmentation (Figure 2.10). These lesions are usually visible except in some heavily coated breeds (e.g. collies) where they may be hidden under the remaining fur. The alopecia may be prominent in short-coated breeds, giving them a moth-eaten appearance (Figure 2.11). Pruritus is variable and is also affected by the underlying cause of the bacterial folliculitis.

Mucocutaneous pyoderma (Figure 2.12) can be seen in any dog, but German shepherd dogs and shepherd mixes may be predisposed (Miller et al. 2013). The cause of mucocutaneous pyoderma is not known and it can occur as a primary disease without any underlying condition. The lesions consist of

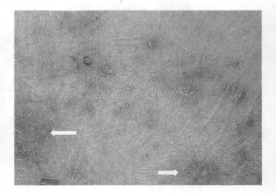

Figure 2.7 Papules (blue arrow) and small epidermal collarettes (white arrows) on the inguinal area of a dog with pyoderma. *Source:* Courtesy of Wayne Rosenkrantz DVM, DACVD, Animal Dermatology Clinic, Tustin, CA.

(a)

(b)

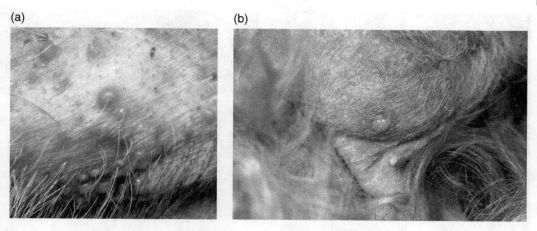

Figure 2.8 (a) Multiple follicular pustules (note hair in the center of several pustules). (b) Single large pustule.

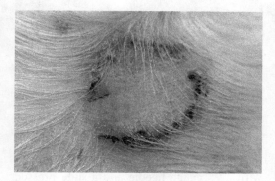

Figure 2.9 Epidermal collarette with circular ring of crusting. Erosion is from skin scraping that was performed.

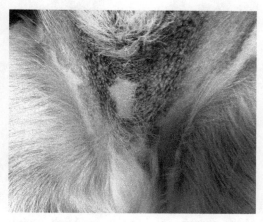

Figure 2.10 Post-inflammatory hyperpigmentation. *Source:* Courtesy of Amy Weller, Dermatology Clinic for Animals, Tacoma, WA.

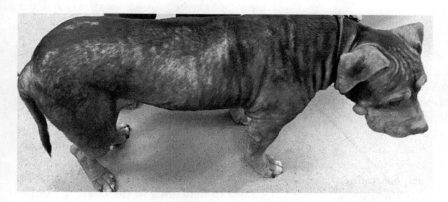

Figure 2.11 Pitbull terrier mix with patchy alopecia resulting in "moth-eaten" appearance.

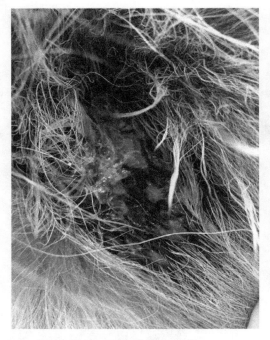

Figure 2.12 Erosions and purulent exudate of mucocutaneous pyoderma in a German shepherd dog.

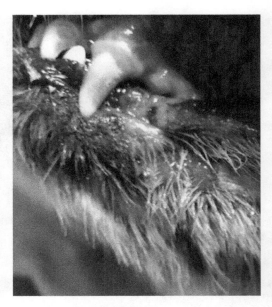

Figure 2.13 Mucocutaneous pyoderma showing affected lip folds and exudate. *Source:* Courtesy of Amy Weller, Dermatology Clinic for Animals, Tacoma, WA.

depigmentation, moist dermatitis, erosion, ulceration, purulent exudate, and crusting. The lips are most commonly affected (Figure 2.13), but lesions can also affect the eyelids, opening of the nares, vulva, opening of the prepuce, and anal area. As the name indicates, lesions can be found anywhere mucous membranes meet epidermis. These lesions can be painful and are sometimes pruritic.

Diagnostic Tests

Patient signalment and clinical signs should be sufficient to make the diagnosis of impetigo. Cytology of pustules can be done to confirm the presence of cocci, but is usually not necessary.

Diagnosis of bacterial folliculitis is also based primarily on history and clinical signs. Cytology of lesions demonstrating the presence of bacteria can confirm the diagnosis, but absence of bacteria on cytology cannot

be used to rule out bacterial folliculitis. Pustule contents and moist exudate under a crust are good samples for cytologic examination. The top of a pustule can be opened with a 25 gauge needle and a slide pressed onto the pustule (see Figures 1.29 and 1.30) or the needle can be used to collect pustule contents and smear them out on a slide. Crusts can be lifted up also with a 25 gauge needle and the slide can be pressed onto the moist skin under the crust. Alternatively, clear tape can be pressed onto the skin under a crust. Slides and tape samples are stained with Diff-Quik and then examined for the presence of bacteria and inflammatory cells. Bacteria should be identified as cocci or rods, and the presence of intracellular bacteria (within neutrophils) should be noted. It is also important to perform deep skin scrapings to look for demodicosis and pluck hair for dermatophyte testing (trichogram, culture, or polymerase chain reaction testing), since these are the other two common causes of folliculitis in the dog. Due to the increased frequency of methicillin-resistant staphylococcal infections, aerobic bacterial culture and sensitivity testing may be needed to guide antibiotic selection for treatment. Indications for culturing include bacterial folliculitis that is not responding to treatment or that is recurrent and has received multiple courses of antibiotic therapy.

The culture can be taken from an intact pustule by opening the surface of the pustule with a 25 gauge needle and dabbing the sterile swab onto the pustule contents. If intact pustules are not present, the sample can be taken from underneath a crust. It is important not to disinfect the area before you acquire your sample, since these are superficial lesions and doing so may affect your culture results.

An effort should be made to determine the underlying cause for the bacterial folliculitis, especially if the folliculitis is a recurrent problem. Historical information including the presence of pruritus, degree and location of pruritus, effect of antibiotic therapy on pruritus, presence or absence of seasonality, flea control measures being used, presence or absence of other affected pets in the household, and degree of contact with other animals outside the household can help determine if allergic disease, ectoparasitism, or endocrine disease is the underlying cause. Physical examination findings will also guide the clinician's search for the underlying cause of the folliculitis.

Treatment

As with surface pyodermas, many cases of mild to moderate superficial pyoderma can be successfully treated with topical therapy. This is particularly true for impetigo, which almost never requires oral antibiotic therapy. Frequent bathing (every one to three days) along with daily use of antibacterial spray, gel, mousse, wipe, or ointment can be very effective. Benzoyl peroxide, chlorhexidine, and ethyl lactate are the most commonly found antibacterial agents in shampoos. Chlorhexidine, benzoyl peroxide, nisin, mupirocin, and other topical antimicrobials are found in a variety of gels, ointments, sprays, wipes, and mousses.

In some cases of severe bacterial folliculitis and most cases of mucocutaneous pyoderma, oral antibiotics are also necessary. Appropriate antibiotics should be given for at least three to four weeks. The current guidelines recommend that all visible lesions should be clear for at least seven days before stopping antibiotics (Hillier et al. 2014). Patients should be re-examined just before finishing antibiotics so the veterinarian can determine if all lesions have truly cleared.

Deep Pyodermas

Deep pyodermas include furunculosis, cellulitis, and panniculitis. Deep pyodermas occur most commonly as an extension of a worsening superficial bacterial folliculitis. The infection causes rupture of the hair follicle and infection of the dermis and subcutaneous tissue. These are more serious infections. Staphylococcal bacteria are most commonly associated with deep pyodermas, but gram-negative bacteria such as *Pseudomonas aeruginosa*, *Proteus mirabilis*, and *E. coli* can also be isolated from these infections fairly frequently. Primary infections of the subcutaneous tissue such as panniculitis caused by *Nocardia sp.* and mycobacterial organisms will not be discussed in this chapter. See the recommended reading list for information on these infections.

Clinical Features

The primary lesion in early deep pyodermas is the furuncle (Figure 2.14). The furuncle is a bulla that contains serosanguinous, hemorrhagic, or purulent exudate. Clients will often describe these lesions as blood blisters or boils. Furuncles are formed when an infected hair follicle ruptures, releasing hair fragments into the surrounding tissue. These hair fragments act as foreign bodies, causing a pronounced inflammatory response. As the

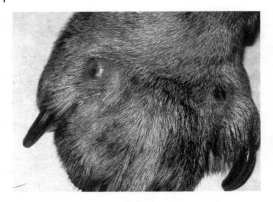

Figure 2.14 Interdigital furunculosis on a front paw of a dog.

disease progresses and more furuncles form, the inflammation coalesces to form firm plaques. As the body continues to try to extrude the hair fragments, draining tracts (see later Figure 2.20) are formed. These lesions are often covered by crusts and matted fur, so clients may be unaware of the extent and severity of their pet's disease.

Furunculosis can be generalized or localized (Figure 2.15). The generalized form of furunculosis is usually a continuation of a superficial pyoderma and can be found on any part of the body. Localized furunculosis

can affect specific areas of the body and cause specific syndromes. Examples of localized furunculosis include acral lick granulomas, muzzle furunculosis, callus pyodermas, interdigital furunculosis, and pyotraumatic folliculitis/furunculosis.

Acral lick granulomas (Figures 2.16 and 2.17) are a common example of localized deep pyoderma secondary to self-trauma and can be seen in any breed of dog. These lesions are mainly found on the distal limbs. They are usually extremely pruritic and consist of a firm nodule with its surface eroded from constant licking. Visible furuncles and draining tracts are present in some but not all cases. Allergies such as atopic dermatitis or food allergy, joint pain from trauma or degenerative joint disease, or behavioral disorders all can cause the initial stimulus for licking.

Muzzle furunculosis (Figure 2.18) is another manifestation of localized deep pyoderma. This is more commonly seen in short-coated breeds with stiff hair coats, such as Doberman pinschers and Labrador retrievers, or in breeds that produce excess saliva, such as mastiffs and English bulldogs (Miller et al. 2013). The lesions initially consist of individual furuncles on the chin and

(a)

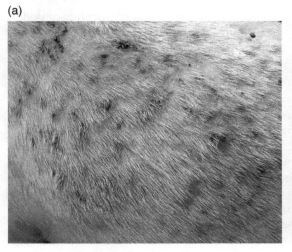

(b)

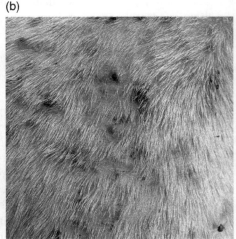

Figure 2.15 (a) Multiple furuncles and crusts on dorsal trunk of a dog. (b) Closer view of the same dog showing hemorrhagic/purulent exudate from ruptured furuncles. *Source:* Courtesy of Nicole A. Boynosky MS, BVMS, DACVD, Veterinary Specialty Hospital, San Diego, CA.

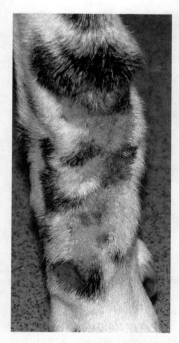

Figure 2.16 Acral lick granuloma on the distal forelimb of a Dalmatian; note alopecia, erythema, and traumatic erosion from licking.

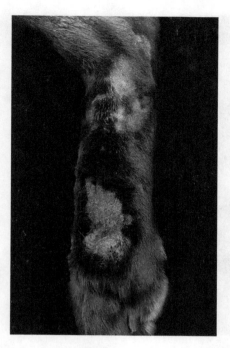

Figure 2.17 Acral lick granuloma on the distal forelimb of a dog. *Source:* Courtesy of Amy Weller, Dermatology Clinic for Animals, Tacoma, WA.

muzzle, but can progress to form firm plaques with or without draining tracts. Many furuncles contain keratinaceous debris or hair fragments that are extruded when the affected area is gently squeezed. These lesions will often heal with pronounced scarring, which can lead to further entrapment of short hairs that perpetuates the inflammation.

Callus pyodermas (Figure 2.19) occur in large-breed dogs that lie down on hard surfaces. The lesions are usually seen on the elbows, hocks, and lateral thighs. As with the other deep pyodermas, they consist of furuncles and draining tracts from which hairs and keratinaceous debris may be expressed.

Interdigital furunculosis is another common form of localized deep pyoderma. It is found most often in short-coated breeds such as boxers, great Danes, or English bulldogs (Miller et al. 2013). It is characterized by large furuncles in the interdigital spaces both dorsally and ventrally. These lesions are usually painful, causing the pet to limp and

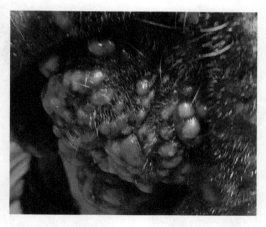

Figure 2.18 Dog with muzzle furunculosis. *Source:* Courtesy of Austin Richman, DVM, DACVD.

lick at them constantly. They tend to rupture on a regular basis, leading to a history of bloody footprints in the home (Figure 2.20). As with muzzle furunculosis, these lesions many times contain small hair fragments and

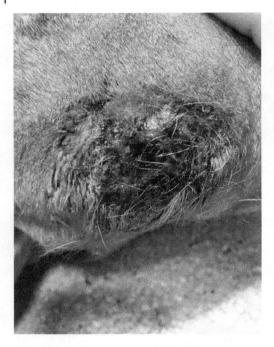

Figure 2.19 Deep callus pyoderma with purulent exudate at a pressure point (elbow). *Source:* Courtesy of Amy Weller, Dermatology Clinic for Animals, Tacoma, WA.

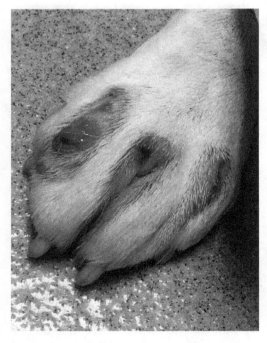

Figure 2.20 Dog with interdigital furuncles and draining tracts.

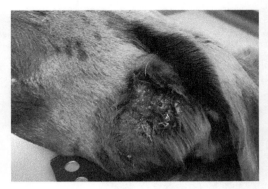

Figure 2.21 Dog with pyotraumatic folliculitis/furunculosis ventral to ear characterized by a firm moist eroded plaque.

keratinaceous debris that can be extruded when the lesion is gently squeezed. These lesions also tend to heal with scarring.

Pyotraumatic folliculitis/furunculosis (Figure 2.21) is another form of localized deep pyoderma. These lesions are often incorrectly diagnosed as acute moist dermatitis, or a "hot spot." True hot spots are surface lesions that occur in areas that the patient can lick or chew and the affected area is not thickened. Pyotraumatic folliculitis/furunculosis is characterized by a firm, moist, eroded plaque ventral to the ear or on the neck, with satellite papules or furuncles that many times cannot be seen until the lesion and surrounding area have been clipped. They can be accompanied by otitis externa, but are not always. Pain and pruritus are variable.

Diagnostic Tests

The diagnosis of deep pyoderma is usually straightforward and can be made from the patient's history and clinical signs. Cytology of exudate from draining tracts or intact furuncles typically shows inflammatory cells (neutrophils, macrophages) and red blood cells. Bacteria are not always visible and their absence does not rule out the diagnosis of deep bacterial infection. Deep pyodermas can require long-term antibiotic therapy, so aerobic culture and sensitivity testing are often indicated. The culture sample should be taken from an intact furuncle if possible. Unlike aerobic culture collection for superficial pyodermas, the skin surface can be cleaned with an antiseptic before a culture is taken. The furuncle is then pierced with a needle and the exudate is collected on a sterile swab. In chronic cases of furunculosis where there is a great deal of scarring, a culture from a tissue biopsy sample may be more likely to reveal the primary causative agent. The biopsy sample for culture should be obtained aseptically and the surface of the skin should be thoroughly disinfected prior to sampling. As with superficial pyodermas, it is important to rule out demodicosis and dermatophytosis, since these are other common primary causes of furunculosis. Additional diagnostic testing to identify underlying causes of the infection may include thyroid hormone measurement, complete blood count, serum biochemistry panel, urinalysis, or other testing as determined by the patient's particular history and clinical signs. If allergic dermatitis is suspected, intensive flea control measures, an elimination diet trial, and finally allergy testing for environmental allergens may be recommended.

Treatment

Deep pyodermas are secondary problems and unless the underlying disease is diagnosed and treated, the deep pyoderma either will not clear or will recur. Most deep pyodermas require long-term systemic antibiotic therapy that should always be based on the results of aerobic culture and sensitivity testing. The length of therapy varies, but should continue for a minimum of six to eight weeks. The surface of the skin will look normal before all deeper lesions have resolved and it is important to make clients aware of this, so they do not stop antibiotic therapy prematurely. In cases with extensive and severe lesions, therapy may be required for many months. Antibiotic therapy should be continued until all lesions have been clear for at least 14 days. In the case of scarred lesions such as acral lick granulomas, the

lesion's improvement should have plateaued for two to three weeks before antibiotic therapy is stopped (Miller et al. 2013).

Frequent bathing and hydrotherapy (soaking) are important treatment modalities for generalized deep pyodermas. Bathing removes crusts, exudate, debris, and bacteria from the skin surface. It also soothes the skin and can decrease pruritus. Chlorhexidine, benzoyl peroxide, and ethyl lactate are the commonly used antibacterial agents in shampoos. Benzoyl peroxide is keratolytic and works to open the follicles, which can help when the infection is deeper in the skin layers. Benzoyl peroxide can also be drying, so chlorhexidine or ethyl lactate may be better tolerated when used multiple times per week.

Topical therapies are also of benefit in treating localized deep pyodermas such as muzzle furunculosis, interdigital furunculosis, and callus pyoderma. All types of localized deep pyodermas benefit from soaking and warm compresses, which help bring the furuncles to a head and flush out the draining tracts. Soaks and compresses can be done with astringents such as Burow's solution or antiseptics such as dilute benzoyl peroxide or chlorhexidine.

Most types of localized deep pyoderma benefit from topical antibiotics. The use of topical antibiotics can sometimes decrease the length of time for which the patient requires systemic antibiotic therapy. It is best if the topical antibiotic is chosen based on the results of culture and sensitivity testing.

Lesions that are lichenified and thickened, such as callus pyodermas and muzzle furunculosis, can also benefit from products that contain keratolytic agents such as benzoyl peroxide, urea, or salicylic acid. It is best to apply these products after the area has been soaked or treated with a wet compress. These products break down the excessive stratum corneum and soften the skin. This allows the hair follicles to open up and function more normally again.

Scarred lesions of muzzle furunculosis and acral lick granulomas may also benefit from topical glucocorticoids that will help break down some of the excess fibrous tissue and decrease the inflammatory response.

Client Education

It is important that clients understand the secondary nature of bacterial skin infections. They will often ask how or where the patient acquired the bacteria, and it is essential to explain that staphylococcal bacteria are normally present on dogs' skin. Clients must understand that these bacteria are normally found in small numbers and that something must disrupt the normal skin surface environment or suppress the patient's immune system to allow the overgrowth of bacteria to occur. Clients must also understand that if the underlying problem is a chronic disease, such as atopic dermatitis or hypothyroidism, the infection will recur if the underlying disease is not diagnosed and treated.

Since topical therapy is important for most bacterial skin infections, clients must be shown good bathing techniques and proper application of topical products. Some owners may not be able to bathe their pets at home. Offering grooming services at the veterinary hospital or having a recommendation for a groomer can be helpful. Bathing can be done indoors or outdoors, depending on facilities and the weather. A secure footing will make pets feel more comfortable, so rubber mats or other non-skid surfacing should be placed into the tub where the pet will be bathed. Patients with long-hair coats may benefit from having the hair clipped short. This allows better visualization of lesions and better contact of shampoo with the skin. Cool to lukewarm water should be used and vigorous scrubbing should be avoided, as warm water and scrubbing can increase non-specific pruritus. If the patient is very dirty, a gentle cleansing shampoo can be used first to remove dirt and debris, then follow with the medicated shampoo. Clients should be warned that medicated shampoos generally do not lather well. They should start the bath by applying shampoo to the most severely affected areas and moving outward from there. A contact time of 10–15 minutes is often recommended. Using toys and treats can help pass the pet's time in the bath and setting a timer can ensure the desired contact time is achieved. Thorough rinsing is also extremely important, as shampoo residue can be irritating. Towel drying is often adequate, but if blow drying is needed only the low heat setting should be used.

Clients should be shown how to apply topical products to the affected areas. Gentle cleaning of skin folds is important for fold pyodermas, both as treatment and for continued preventative care. Cleaning and treatment can be done with antimicrobial wipes, or wipes can be followed by application of another product. For all topical products, it is important that patients do not remove the medication by licking it off. This can be accomplished by the use of Elizabethan collars or clothing that covers the affected area until the medication is absorbed into the skin. Another option is to distract patients by playing with them or taking them for a walk immediately after product application.

Good antibiotic stewardship is more important than ever due to the increased incidence of multi-drug-resistant staphylococcal infections (Hillier et al. 2014). Giving oral antibiotics at the correct dose at the prescribed interval for the entire length of time recommended must be emphasized to clients. The veterinary staff must ensure that the client is able to administer the antibiotic in the form prescribed (pill or capsule or liquid) and at the prescribed frequency. Once to twice to three times a day administration may be needed. A recheck appointment should be scheduled just before the antibiotic course is finished so the clinician can determine if the infection has cleared completely. Clients should be advised that they should continue antibiotics until their recheck, even if the skin looks clear to them before this time. This is particularly important for deep pyodermas that can require multiple months of antibiotic therapy. Owners should be made aware of possible side effects of the antibiotic and encouraged to call if they are having any problems giving the medication or are seeing any side effects of the medication.

Feline Bacterial Skin Infections

With the exception of subcutaneous abscesses caused by bite wounds, bacterial skin infections are rare in cats. As in the dog, most of these infections are a secondary problem and the underlying cause must be addressed to avoid recurrent infections. *S. aureus* and *S. pseudintermedius* are the staphylococcal bacteria most commonly isolated from bacterial skin infections in cats (Miller et al. 2013; Noli and Morris 2012). Surface infection of eroded or ulcerated lesions such as eosinophilic plaques, eosinophilic granulomas, and excoriations secondary to allergic skin disease is not unusual (Miller et al. 2013; Noli and Morris 2012). Surface cytology from these lesions demonstrating the presence of cocci can confirm bacterial infection.

Localized lesions (Figure 2.22) can be treated with antibacterial sprays, gels, wipes, or mousses. Cats may not tolerate sprays, so applying the spray to a cotton pad and then wiping it on the lesion may work better.

Because most cats will groom off topical medications, Elizabethan collars or clothing should be used as a barrier after medication is applied.

Superficial bacterial folliculitis in the cat is rare and when present may be associated with underlying systemic illnesses such as feline immunodeficiency virus infection, feline leukemia virus infection, diabetes mellitus, or hyperadrenocorticism (Noli and Morris 2012). Multiple small crusted papules (miliary dermatitis) are the most common clinical presentation of superficial bacterial folliculitis in the cat, and must be differentiated from all the other causes of miliary dermatitis. These include parasitic infestations, fungal skin infections, and allergic diseases. Antibacterial shampooing can be beneficial if the cat is able to be bathed; however, systemic antibiotic therapy is often required, since many cats cannot be easily bathed.

The most common form of deep pyoderma in the cat is bacterial infection of chin acne lesions (Miller et al. 2013; Noli and Morris 2012). Feline chin acne is a keratinization defect that causes dilated, keratin-filled hair follicles (comedones) to form on the chin (Figure 2.23). When these follicles become infected, erythema, swelling, furuncles, and draining tracts form (Figure 2.24). These lesions can be pruritic and painful. Topical therapy with warm compresses and 2% mupirocin antibiotic ointment will successfully

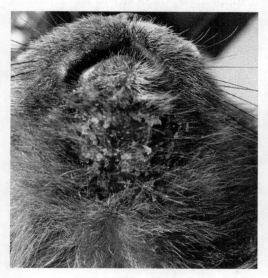

Figure 2.22 Bacterial infection in a cat with a crusty and alopecic chin. *Source:* Courtesy of Amy Weller, Dermatology Clinic for Animals, Tacoma, WA.

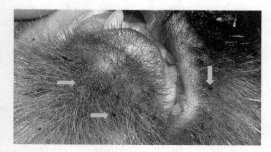

Figure 2.23 Cat with mild chin acne showing comedones (keratin-filled hair follicles). Arrows indicate some of several comedones. *Source:* Courtesy of Dr. Sheila Torres, University of Minnesota.

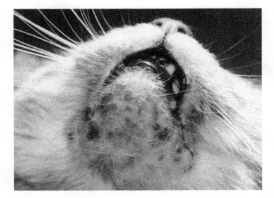

Figure 2.24 Cat with severe chin acne showing furuncles. *Source:* Courtesy of Nellie Choi, BVMS, Dip ACVD, Animal Dermatology Clinic, Perth, Australia.

resolve many cases. On rare occasions, oral antibiotics and corticosteroids may be needed.

Skin infections caused by other bacteria such as *Actinomyces spp.*, *Nocardia spp.*, and mycobacterial organisms are even less common and will not be discussed here. See the recommended reading list for information on these infections.

Methicillin-Resistant Staphylococcal Infections

Over the last 10–15 years, veterinary medicine has seen an alarming increase in the number of methicillin-resistant staphylococcal infections in dogs and cats. These infections do not differ in clinical appearance or severity from those caused by methicillin-sensitive staphylococci, but their treatment is much more challenging. Because they do not differ clinically, the only way to diagnose a resistant infection is via bacterial culture and sensitivity testing. Patients with recurrent or chronic skin infections who have received multiple courses of antibiotics are at increased risk for methicillin-resistant staphylococcal infections. These patients as well as those who are not responding to empirically chosen antibiotic therapy should be cultured and antibiotic selection for these patients will

be based on culture and sensitivity testing results. More recently, increased emphasis is being placed on topical therapy for bacterial skin infections in order to decrease the use of systemic antibiotics. Identifying and treating the underlying cause of the bacterial skin infection is even more important for patients with methicillin-resistant staphylococcal infections.

The zoonotic risk for *S. pseudintermedius* is very low, as this bacterium does not transfer easily to humans (http://www.wormsandgermsblog.com/files/2008/04/JSW-MA3-MRSP-Owner.pdf). Immunosuppressed individuals, for example cancer patients, patients on immunosuppressive drug therapy, and the very young or old, will be at increased risk for infection. Good hygiene should always be recommended. This means washing hands or using alcohol-based hand sanitizers before and after touching pets, avoiding contact with pets' mouths and tongues, and keeping infected areas of skin covered when practical.

When methicillin-resistant *Staphylococcus aureus* (MRSA) is cultured from a dog or a cat, it is important to remember that a human in the household may be the source of the bacteria. MRSA strains are found both in hospitals and in the community at large. Owners should be asked if anyone in the household has been diagnosed with an MRSA infection or is a health-care worker or has been hospitalized recently. Therapy dogs that visit hospitals or nursing homes would also be considered at increased risk for exposure to MRSA. Greater emphasis should be placed on good hygiene practices in cases of MRSA infections in dogs and cats, since *S. aureus* can be passed back from the pet to people (http://www.wormsandgermsblog.com/files/2008/04/M2-MRSA-Owner.pdf).

Preventing the spread of methicillin-resistant staphylococci in the veterinary hospital requires the effort of the entire staff. All hospitals should have an infection control program that addresses all infectious diseases, including staphylococcal infections

(Canadian Committee on Antibiotic Resistance 2008; Weese 2012). Patients with known methicillin-resistant staphylococcal infections should be isolated from the general population and personal protective equipment, including gloves and lab coats or other protective clothing, should be worn when handling these pets. All surfaces and equipment these patients contact should be thoroughly cleaned and disinfected. Since bacterial culture and sensitivity testing are required to identify methicillin-resistant staphylococcal infections, each hospital will need to decide the relative risk for each of its dermatological patients and determine the appropriate infection control procedures. As a general rule, all veterinary staff should sanitize their hands before and after touching patients, even if gloves are worn during patient contact. Hand hygiene can be accomplished by washing with soap and water or by using alcohol-based hand sanitizers. Alcohol-based hand sanitizers are usually more convenient, but if hands are visibly soiled, they should be washed first with soap and water prior to applying the hand sanitizer. Surfaces such as scales, exam tables, and exam room floors (if necessary) should be cleaned and disinfected between each patient. Be sure the disinfectant being used is effective against staphylococcal organisms. Consideration should also be given to isolating immunocompromised patients from the rest of the hospital population, since they will be at increased risk for infection.

Conclusion

Bacterial skin infections are a common problem in canine patients. Understanding that these infections are a secondary phenomenon is crucial for proper treatment of the infection as well as prevention of future infections. Educating and informing clients will not only help bring comfort to the patient, but will also prevent owner frustration. Setting appropriate expectations about the length and type of therapy required, as well as explaining the reason for recheck appointments, is also important. Most clients want to be actively involved in their pet's treatment, and the veterinary staff must listen to and address their concerns as early as possible. Periodic phone calls to check on a patient's progress and to answer any questions clients may have can help ensure a successful outcome for the patient.

References

Canadian Committee on Antibiotic Resistance (2008). Infection prevention and control best practices. Ontario: CCAR-CCRA. http://www.wormsandgermsblog.com/files/2008/04/CCAR-Guidelines-Final2.pdf (accessed November 2015).

Hillier, A., Lloyd, D.H., Weese, J.S. et al. (2014). Guidelines for the diagnosis and antimicrobial therapy of superficial bacterial folliculitis (Antimicrobial Guidelines Working Group of the International Society for Companion Animal Infectious Diseases). *Veterinary Dermatology* 25: 163–e43.

Miller, W.H., Griffin, C.E., and Campbell, K.L. (2013). *Muller and Kirk's Small Animal Dermatology*, 7e. St. Louis, Missouri: Elsevier.

Noli, C. and Morris, D.O. (2012). Staphylococcal pyoderma. In: *BSAVA Manual of Canine and Feline Dermatology*, 3e (eds. H.A. Jackson and R. Marsella), 183–187. Gloucester, UK: BSAVA.

Weese, J.S. (2012). Staphylococcal control in the veterinary hospital. *Veterinary Dermatology* 23: 292–300.

MRSP for pet owners. *Worms & Germs Blog*, May 16, 2011. http://www.wormsandgermsblog.com/files/2008/04/JSW-MA3-MRSP-Owner.pdf (accessed November 2015).

MRSA for pet owners. *Worms & Germs Blog*, September 28, 2008. http://www.wormsandgermsblog.com/files/2008/04/M2-MRSA-Owner.pdf (accessed November 2015).

Recommended Reading

Centers for Disease Control and Prevention (2016). When and how to wash your hands. http://www.cdc.gov/handwashing/when-how-handwashing.html (accessed November 2015).

Federation of European Companion Animal Veterinary Associations (2014). FECAVA key recommendations for hygiene and infection control in veterinary practice. http://www.fecava.org/sites/default/files/files/2014_12_recommandation_hygiene.pdf (accessed November 2015).

Miller, W., Griffin, C., and Campbell, K. (2012). *Muller and Kirk's Small Animal Dermatology*, 7e. Philadelphia, PA: Saunders.

Sykes, J. and Greene, C. (2011). *Greene's Infectious Diseases of the Dog and Cat*, 4e. Philadelphia, PA: Saunders.

3

Malassezia Dermatitis

Barbara Haimbach

Introduction

Malassezia yeasts are commensal organisms that make up part of the normal skin microbiome of dogs and cats. They are often found in small numbers on mucocutaneous junctions (lips, anus, vagina, prepuce), interdigital skin, and in the ear canals of dogs and cats (Nuttall 2012). *Malassezia pachydermatis* is the lipophilic but non-lipid-dependent species found on dogs. Cats are most often colonized by *M. pachydermatis*, but other lipid-dependent yeast species including *Malassezia sympodialis, Malassezia furfur, Malassezia slooffiae,* and *Malassezia nana* may also be found (Bond 2012). Any disruption of the skin's microenvironment or immunological defenses can result in *Malassezia* overgrowth and infection. Allergic dermatitis, endocrinopathies, systemic illness, keratinization defects, and excessive skin folds can all be associated with *Malassezia* dermatitis. *Malassezia* dermatitis often occurs together with staphylococcal pyodermas and these microorganisms may have a symbiotic relationship (Miller et al. 2013; Nuttall 2012). Hypersensitivity reactions to *Malassezia* antigens have been demonstrated in some atopic dogs and might explain some dogs' severe clinical signs without cytological evidence of increased numbers of *Malassezia* organisms (Morris 2014; Nuttall 2012).

M. pachydermatis can temporarily colonize human skin and infections of immunocompromised individuals have been reported; therefore, owners of pets with *Malassezia* dermatitis should be counseled on good hand hygiene (Miller et al. 2013; Nuttall 2012).

Clinical Features (Canine)

Malassezia dermatitis is common in dogs and can be seen in any age, sex, or breed. Those breeds that seem to be predisposed include American cocker spaniels, Australian and silky terriers, basset hounds, boxers, Cavalier King Charles spaniels, dachshunds, English setters, German shepherd dogs, Shih tzus, and toy and miniature poodles (Miller et al. 2013). *Malassezia* dermatitis can be localized or generalized (Figures 3.1 and 3.2). Commonly affected areas include ears (see Chapter 4), lips, muzzle, ventral neck, axillae, inguinal area, medial thighs, feet, perianal skin, and skin folds (Miller et al. 2013; Nuttall 2012). Pruritus is almost always present and can be intense. Early lesions consist of erythema, papules, greasy or waxy exudate on the skin (Figure 3.3), and crusting or scaling. With time, the skin can become alopecic, lichenified, and hyperpigmented (Figure 3.4). These patients often have a musty or rancid smell. Dogs with

Small Animal Dermatology for Technicians and Nurses, First Edition. Edited by Kim Horne, Marcia Schwassmann and Dawn Logas.

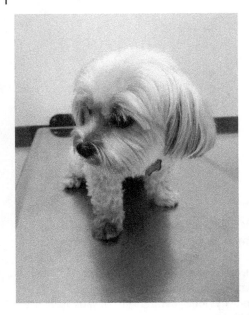

Figure 3.1 Dog with localized *Malassezia* dermatitis affecting the right front foot.

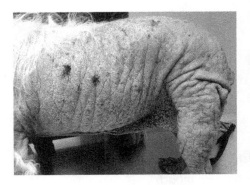

Figure 3.2 Dog with generalized *Malassezia* dermatitis showing alopecia, lichenification, and hyperpigmentation. *Source:* Courtesy of Dr. Brian Palmeiro.

Malassezia pododermatitis can show brown discoloration of paw fur (Figure 3.5) and dogs with *Malassezia* paronychia can have brown discoloration and waxy brown exudate on the nails (Figure 3.6) (Bond 2012; Miller et al. 2013; Nuttall 2012).

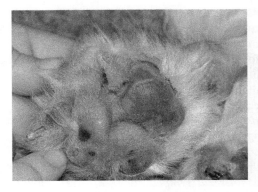

Figure 3.3 Dog with interdigital erythematous, waxy lesion on foot.

(a)

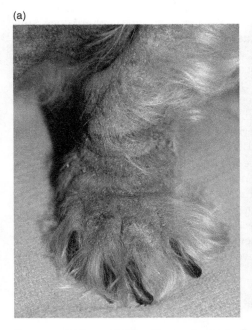

(b)

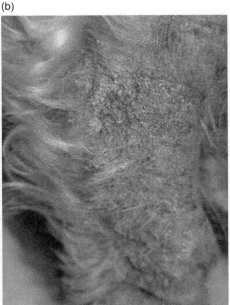

Figure 3.4 (a) Dog with lichenification, hyperpigmentation, and crusting of leg. (b) Close-up view of the same dog.

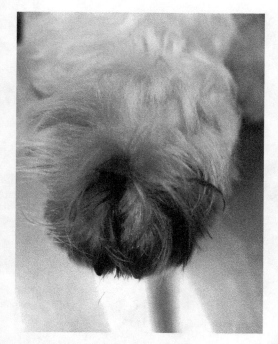

Figure 3.5 Brown discoloration of paw fur on a dog with *Malassezia* pododermatitis (close-up of the dog in Figure 3.1).

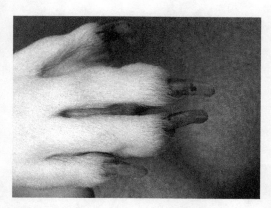

Figure 3.6 Dog with *Malassezia* paronychia showing brown discoloration and waxy brown exudate on the nails. *Source:* Courtesy of Dr. Brian Palmeiro.

Clinical Features (Feline)

Malassezia dermatitis is less common in cats and pruritus is not always present. Devon Rex cats may be predisposed to *Malassezia* paronychia and generalized *Malassezia* dermatitis (Miller et al. 2013; Nuttall 2012).

No other breed, age, or sex predilections have been reported. The disease can be localized (Figure 3.7) or generalized. Cats can present with chin acne or paronychia and brachycephalic breeds such as Persians and Himalayans may present with facial dermatitis (dark crusting and follicular casts; Figure 3.8). Generalized *Malassezia* dermatitis has been reported in association with feline immunodeficiency virus infection, thymoma, paraneoplastic alopecia due to pancreatic adenocarcinoma, and allergic dermatitis (Miller et al. 2013; Nuttall 2012; Ordeix et al. 2007). Cats with generalized disease usually present with erythema, scaling, and some degree of alopecia. Waxy brown exudate on the nails is typically seen in cases of *Malassezia* paronychia (Figure 3.9).

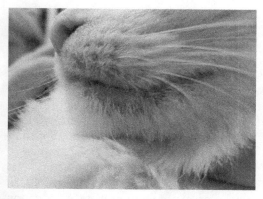

Figure 3.7 Cat with localized *Malassezia* dermatitis affecting lip fold.

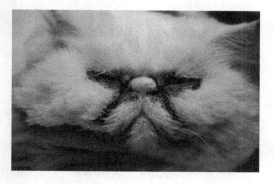

Figure 3.8 Persian cat showing facial dermatitis with dark crusting. *Source:* Photo by Dr. Sheila Torres, courtesy of the University of Minnesota, College of Veterinary Medicine.

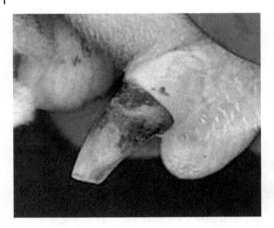

Figure 3.9 Brown nail bed exudate from a domestic short-hair cat with chronic *Malassezia* dermatitis. *Source:* Courtesy of Judy K Lethbridge, CVT, Veterinary Dermatology Center, Maitland, FL.

Diagnostic Tests

Malassezia dermatitis cannot be diagnosed based on appearance alone, since its clinical signs can be very similar to other infectious and allergic skin disorders, such as superficial pyoderma, food allergy, or atopic dermatitis. The most accurate and easiest way to identify *Malassezia* organisms is by skin cytology. Various sample collection methods are commonly used. A plain glass slide can be pressed onto the skin for a direct impression. This method is most useful for flat areas of skin that have waxy or moist exudate. A dry cotton swab can be vigorously rubbed on the skin surface, again preferably on an area that has moist or waxy exudate, and then rolled onto a glass slide. For areas that are drier, a spatula or dull scalpel blade can be used to lightly scrape the surface of the skin and the collected material can be smeared onto a glass slide. Alternatively, a thin strip of clear packing tape (e.g. Scotch® heavy duty shipping tape) can be pressed repeatedly onto the skin surface. Sampling with a toothpick proved superior to tape impressions and direct impressions of nail folds (Lo and Rosenkrantz 2016). Slides or tape strips can be stained with Diff-Quik (see Chapter 1 for more details on how to obtain and prepare skin cytology samples).

Alternatively, a drop of new methylene blue stain or the purple stain from the Diff-Quik set can be used alone. This method produces a monochrome image that beginners may find more difficult to evaluate. Microscopically, *Malassezia* are small, oval to peanut or snowman shaped organisms (Figures 3.10 and 3.11). They typically stain a dark blue, but can sometimes be reddish-pink or pale blue (Nuttall 2012). There is no uniformly accepted number of yeast organisms required to diagnose *Malassezia* dermatitis. Normal yeast numbers can vary between breeds as well as body sites. As a general rule, cytology from normal skin only occasionally shows *Malassezia* organisms. Various numbers

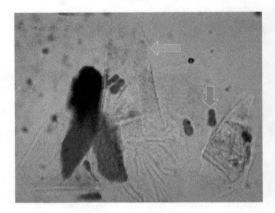

Figure 3.10 Microscopic image of epithelial cells (orange arrow) and *Malassezia* organisms (blue arrow).

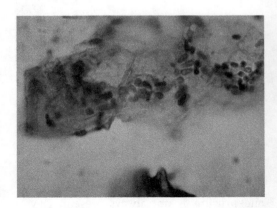

Figure 3.11 Microscopic image of *Malassezia* organisms.

ranging from greater than 2 organisms per oil power field (x1000) to greater than 10 organisms per oil power field have been proposed as diagnostic (Miller et al. 2013; Nuttall 2012). Some dogs develop a yeast hypersensitivity, so even if only a few yeast are found on cytology, treatment may still be indicated.

Yeast organisms may also be seen on biopsy samples taken for histopathology. Since *Malassezia* organisms are found in the outer layers of the stratum corneum and in the hair follicles, they are sometimes removed and lost during sample processing (Miller et al. 2013, Nuttall 2012). Cultures are not useful for diagnosis, since *Malassezia* yeasts are present on normal skin. *Malassezia* hypersensitivity can now be assessed by intradermal testing and by measurement of serum immunoglobulin E (IgE) levels. The value of the diagnostic testing and immunotherapy with *Malassezia* extracts is not universally accepted, but preliminary studies are promising (Aberg et al. 2017; Farver et al. 2005; Morris 2014; Oldenhoff et al. 2014).

The diagnosis of *Malassezia* dermatitis ultimately is confirmed when a patient responds to antifungal treatment.

Treatment

The goal of treatment for *Malassezia* dermatitis is twofold: first to control the current infection, and second to identify and treat the underlying disease(s). If an underlying cause cannot be found or effectively managed, recurrence of the infection is likely and lifetime maintenance therapy may be required.

Malassezia dermatitis can be treated topically, systemically, or with a combination of both. The type of treatment is determined by the area(s) affected, the severity of infection and clinical signs, patient factors, and the capabilities of the client to administer the recommended treatment. Topical therapy is often the least expensive and safest, but is the most labor intensive. Clients may be unwilling or unable to comply with topical therapy

recommendations. To ensure compliance, therapeutic options must be discussed with the client to determine the best treatment plan for each individual patient and owner.

Patients with either localized or multifocal *Malassezia* dermatitis will benefit from topical therapy. Bathing at least twice a week with an antifungal shampoo and a 10-minute contact time is recommended (Miller et al. 2013). Cool to lukewarm water is best, as it can help decrease inflammation and irritation and reduce the level of pruritus. Concentrate on those areas of the body that are clinically most affected, as well as areas more likely to have increased numbers of yeast organisms, such as the feet, ventral neck, lip folds, axillae, and inguinal area (Nuttall 2012). Since yeast organisms thrive best in moist, warm environments, thoroughly drying the pet afterwards is also important. Many antifungal shampoos are available for veterinary use. These products contain one or more antifungal agents such as chlorhexidine, climbazole, ketoconazole, and miconazole. Reviews of the literature found good evidence for the efficacy of a 2% chlorhexidine 2% miconazole shampoo when used twice a week for three weeks (Mueller et al. 2012; Negre et al. 2009). Many of these agents are also available in other formulations, such as wipes, rinses, mousses, and sprays for spot treatment or generalized application. These topical antifungals are generally well tolerated and irritant reactions are rare. Other less commonly used topical antifungals include 2% lime sulfur dip (not available in Europe), 0.2% enilconazole rinse (not available in the United States), 1% selenium sulfide shampoo (dogs only), and 2.5% acetic acid rinse (Miller et al. 2013). If a patient has moderate to severe disease or recurring infection, or if it is difficult for the owner to bathe their pet, it may be better to utilize systemic antifungal therapy. Currently available oral antifungal agents include fluconazole, itraconazole, ketoconazole, and terbinafine. None of these drugs is label approved in the United States for the treatment of *Malassezia* dermatitis in dogs and cats.

Ketoconazole is generally well tolerated in dogs. Adverse effects are uncommon, but gastrointestinal upset (inappetence, vomiting, diarrhea) and rare hepatotoxicity can be seen. Ketoconazole should not be used in cats due to the high incidence of adverse effects, including weight loss, anorexia, vomiting, and hepatotoxicity. The recommended dose is 5–10 mg/kg once a day for three to four weeks, and it is best absorbed when given with food. Ketoconazole interacts with many other drugs, so a complete list of other medications the patient is taking should be obtained before starting therapy (Miller et al. 2013).

Itraconazole given at 5 mg/kg daily for three weeks has good efficacy against *Malassezia* dermatitis and can be used in dogs and cats. Adverse effects are less frequent and drug interactions are fewer than with ketoconazole, but the expense of this drug may limit its use in veterinary medicine (Miller et al. 2013). Because itraconazole accumulates in the skin, pulse dosing (given on two consecutive days per week) has also been successful (Pinchbeck et al. 2002). Itraconazole is best absorbed in the presence of food. The compounded formulations of this medication should not be used due to inadequate absorption from the gastrointestinal tract (Mawby et al. 2014).

Fluconazole is given at 5–10 mg/kg daily for both dogs and cats. Efficacy was shown to be equivalent to ketoconazole in dogs with *Malassezia* dermatitis (Sickafoose et al. 2010). This drug is eliminated primarily by renal excretion. Adverse effects and hepatotoxicity are seen less often than with ketoconazole and itraconazole.

Terbinafine is being used more commonly as treatment for *Malassezia* dermatitis in dogs and for treatment of dermatophytosis in cats. A pilot study demonstrated good efficacy at a dose of 30 mg/kg daily or twice a week, but further studies are needed to confirm its effectiveness (Berger et al. 2012). This drug is best absorbed when given with food and has few drug interactions (Miller et al. 2013). Some clinicians routinely monitor liver enzymes before and during therapy with oral antifungals due to the potential for hepatotoxicity with some of these medications.

Patients should always be rechecked toward the end of their treatment. A combination of systemic and topical therapy should provide the quickest clinical improvement, followed by systemic therapy, and then topical therapy. Cytology samples should be evaluated at each recheck. These results, along with clinical response to therapy, will determine if the infection has resolved or if longer treatment is necessary. Ideally, therapy should be continued for 7–10 days after clinical resolution (Miller et al. 2013).

Patients with recurrent *Malassezia* dermatitis may benefit from regular bathing with antifungal shampoos. This can help reduce the numbers of yeast organisms on the skin and might prevent or at least decrease recurrent infections. Pulse dosing of oral antifungal drugs may be required for patients who fail to respond to maintenance topical therapy.

Client Education

The veterinary technician is often responsible for obtaining the medical history for patients. This information can provide important clues to the identification of the underlying cause of *Malassezia* dermatitis. Having the owner complete a dermatology questionnaire (see example in Chapter 1) prior to their appointment is helpful. Important questions to ask include what clinical signs the patient is exhibiting, whether this is the first time this problem has occurred or is it a recurrent problem, at what age clinical signs first began, if this is a chronic problem have clinical signs changed over time, is the problem seasonal or year round, is the patient pruritic and if yes how severe the pruritus is, what treatments have been used and what has been the response to treatment, does the patient have any other medical problems, and does the patient have any other signs of illness (e.g. vomiting, diarrhea, increased drinking or urination).

A complete list of current medications, both systemic and topical, should be obtained.

The veterinary technician will most likely be the person responsible for explaining the treatment plan to the owner. Ensuring the client understands the recommended treatment plan as well as how to administer and apply medications will help the client to be successful and should improve compliance. It is important to teach clients proper bathing and ear cleaning techniques, how to properly apply topical medications, and how to keep the pet from licking off these medications. *Malassezia* infections will not resolve overnight, so it is imperative that the client understands the importance of following the treatment protocol as instructed for the entire treatment period recommended. It is also vital to counsel owners regarding what to expect from therapy. For example, patients with atopic dermatitis may continue to develop secondary bacterial and/or yeast infections while waiting for their allergen-specific immunotherapy to start working. If clients understand the secondary nature of *Malassezia* dermatitis, they will be more likely to follow recommendations regarding treating the underlying cause of the infection. The importance of recheck examinations must also be stressed. Cytology can confirm resolution of infection or can show residual yeast organisms that might indicate the need for maintenance antifungal therapy. The veterinary technician is also responsible for a good portion of follow-up client communication. Calling the client periodically during the treatment period to find out how the pet is doing, ensuring medications are being administered correctly, and reporting any problems to the veterinarian can be helpful in the management of these cases.

Conclusion

Many patients with *Malassezia* dermatitis will respond favorably to therapy. Once the underlying cause is identified and managed, infections with *Malassezia* yeast should become less frequent or stop altogether. However, if an underlying cause is not diagnosed and treated, it is likely that infections will be recurrent and lifelong maintenance therapy may be needed. This can be very frustrating for both the owner as well as the veterinary staff. Being supportive, compassionate, and understanding will not only help owners, but will also make it easier for them to help their pets.

References

Aberg, L., Varjonen, K., and Ahman, S. (2017). Results of allergen-specific immunotherapy in atopic dogs with *Malassezia* hypersensitivity: a retrospective study of 16 cases. *Veterinary Dermatology* 28 (6): 633–e157.

Berger, D.J., Lewis, T.P., Schick, A.E., and Stone, R.T. (2012). Comparison of once-daily versus twice-weekly terbinafine administrations for the treatment of canine *Malassezia* dermatitis- a pilot study. *Veterinary Dermatology* 23 (5): 418–e79.

Bond, R. (2012). Malassezia dermatitis. In: *Infectious Diseases of the Dog and Cat*, 4e (ed. C.E. Greene), 602–606. Elsevier Saunders.

Farver, K., Morris, D.O., Shofer, F., and Esch, B. (2005). Humoral measurement of type-1 hypersensitivity reactions to a commercial Malassezia antigen. *Veterinary Dermatology* 16 (4): 261–268.

Lo, K.L. and Rosenkrantz, W.S. (2016). Evaluation of cytology collection techniques and prevalence of *Malassezia* yeast and bacteria in claw folds of normal and allergic dogs. *Veterinary Dermatology* 27 (4): 279–e67.

Mawby, D.I., Whittemore, J.C., Genger, S., and Papich, M.G. (2014). Bioequivalence of orally administered generic, compounded, and innovato-formulated itraconazole in healthy dogs. *Journal of Veterinary Internal Medicine* 28 (1): 72–77.

Miller, W.H., Griffin, C.E., and Campbell, K.L. (2013). Fungal and algal skin diseases. In: *Muller & Kirk's Small Animal Dermatology*, 7e, 223–283. St. Louis: Elsevier Mosby.

Morris, D.O. (2014). Malassezia infections. In: *Kirk's Current Veterinary Therapy XV* (eds. J.D. Bonagura and D.C. Twedt), e212–e216. Philadelphia, PA: Saunders.

Mueller, R.S., Bergvall, K., Bensignor, E., and Bond, R. (2012). A review of topical therapy for skin infections with bacteria and yeast. *Veterinary Dermatology* 23 (4): 330–e62.

Negre, A., Bensignor, E., and Guillot, J. (2009). Evidence-based veterinary dermatology: a systematic review of interventions for *Malassezia* dermatitis in dogs. *Veterinary Dermatology* 20 (1): 1–12.

Nuttall, T. (2012). Malassezia dermatitis. In: *BSAVA Manual of Small Animal Dermatology, Third Edition* (eds. H. Jackson and R. Marsella), 198–205. British Small Animal Veterinary Association.

Oldenhoff, W.E., Frank, G.R., and DeBoer, D.J. (2014). Comparison of results of intradermal test reactivity and serum allergen-specific IgE measurement for *Malassezia pachydermatis* in atopic dogs. *Veterinary Dermatology* 25 (6): 507–e85.

Ordeix, L., Galeotti, F., Scarampella, F. et al. (2007). *Malassezia* spp. overgrowth in allergic cats. *Veterinary Dermatology* 18 (5): 316–323.

Pinchbeck, L., Hillier, A., Kowalski, J., and Kwochka, K. (2002). Comparison of pulse administration versus once daily administration of itraconazole for the treatment of *Malassezia pachydermatis* dermatitis and otitis in dogs. *Journal of the American Veterinary Medical Association* 220 (12): 1807–1812.

Sickafoose, L., Hosgood, G., Snook et al. (2010). A noninferiority clinical trial comparing fluconazole and ketoconazole in combination with cephalexin for the treatment of dogs with Malassezia dermatitis. *Veterinary Therapeutics* 11 (2): E1–E13.

4

Otitis Externa

Dawn Logas

Introduction

Otitis externa in dogs is seen on a regular basis in clinical practice. According to data from Nationwide®, a large provider of veterinary pet insurance in the United States, it was the second most common medical condition reported for dogs in 2018 (Nationwide 2018). Otodectic acariasis (ear mites) is common in kittens, but in general otitis externa is seen less frequently in cats. It is important to understand that otitis externa simply means inflammation of the external ear canal. This inflammation has a variety of causes and is often complicated by infection with bacterial or yeast organisms. Otitis externa is more accurately considered a sign of another problem rather than a stand-alone disease. It is therefore important not only to treat any active infection that may be present, but also to investigate the underlying cause of the inflammation. Complete treatment for otitis externa that addresses primary causes as well as secondary microbial infection results in healthier patients and happier owners.

Pathogenesis

The canine and feline ear is divided into three parts (Figure 4.1). The external ear canal extends from its opening at the base of the ear pinna proximally through the vertical and horizontal canals to the tympanic membrane. The tympanic membrane separates the middle ear cavity from the external ear canal. The middle ear cavity consists of the tympanic bulla and the auditory ossicles (malleus, incus, and stapes). In cats, an almost complete bony septum divides the tympanic bulla into two parts (Bensignor and Forsythe 2012). The inner ear contains the semicircular canals that are responsible for balance and the cochlea that is responsible for hearing. The external ear canal is lined by epithelium along with its normal adnexal structures, including hair follicles, ceruminous glands, and sebaceous glands. The ear has a self-cleaning mechanism that is based on epithelial cell migration. Epithelial cells move outward from the center of the tympanic membrane, then distally along the wall of the ear canal, carrying debris and cerumen out of the external ear canal and keeping it clean (Miller et al. 2013).

The causes of otitis externa have been divided into three categories: predisposing factors, primary causes, and perpetuating factors (Bensignor and Forsythe 2012; Miller et al. 2013). All three of these must be addressed to successfully treat otitis externa and prevent frequent relapses. Predisposing factors alter the microenvironment of the ear canal to make it more favorable for the development of otitis externa. Predisposing factors include environmental conditions, anatomic variations of the ear canal, and any systemic disease that compromises immune

Small Animal Dermatology for Technicians and Nurses, First Edition. Edited by Kim Horne, Marcia Schwassmann and Dawn Logas.
© 2020 John Wiley & Sons, Inc. Published 2020 by John Wiley & Sons, Inc.

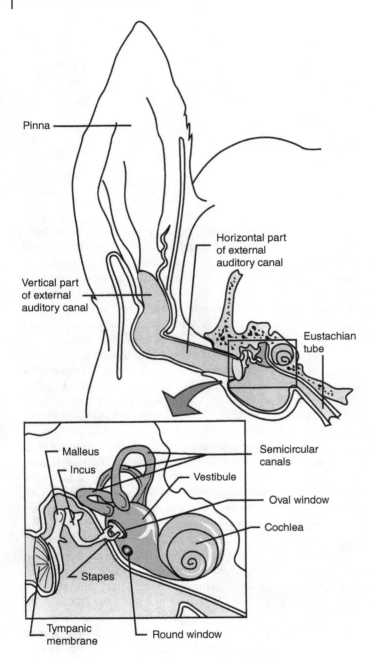

Figure 4.1 Diagram of canine ear. *Source:* T. Colville and J.M. Bassert (2016). *Sense Organs in Clinical Anatomy and Physiology for Veterinary Technicians*, 3rd edn. Figure 10.4 Cross section of dog's ear structures with middle and inner ear regions enlarged, p. 261. Reproduced with permission of Elsevier. © Elsevier 2016.

system function. Otitis externa is more common in warm, humid climates, and frequent bathing or swimming can also increase humidity in the ear canal. There are both gross and microscopic anatomical variations that predispose different breeds to otitis externa. Some breeds of dogs with pendulous ears have significantly more otitis externa than breeds with erect ear pinnae, perhaps due to increased humidity within the ear canal. Most Chinese shar peis have congenitally narrow vertical canals that predispose them to chronic otitis externa. Certain breeds of dogs such as cocker spaniels, springer spaniels, and Labrador retrievers have more ceruminous or wax glands in their horizontal ear canals that increase their chances of developing otitis externa. Breeds that have an increased number of hairs in the horizontal canal, such as poodles, can also be predisposed to otitis externa.

Primary causes of otitis externa are diseases that by themselves directly cause inflammation of the ear canal. These include parasites (*Otodectes cynotis, Demodex canis, Demodex cati, Sarcoptes scabiei*), foreign bodies such as plant awns, tumors, and keratinization disorders such as hypothyroidism (Figures 4.2 and 4.3). But by far the most common primary cause of bilateral otitis externa in the dog is allergic dermatitis, in particular atopic dermatitis and food allergy. The majority of dogs with food allergy or atopic dermatitis have otitis externa as part of their clinical signs, and in a small number of dogs it is the only consistent sign they exhibit.

Perpetuating factors are a consequence of the inflammation and if left untreated, can

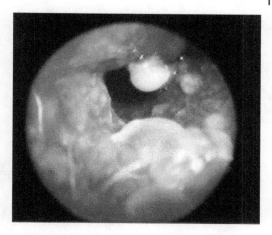

Figure 4.3 Video-otoscopic picture of small mass in ear.

prevent the resolution of or worsen an already existing otitis externa. Examples of perpetuating factors include infectious agents such as bacteria and yeast, otitis media, chronic pathological changes of the ear canal, and iatrogenic causes such as contact reactions to medications and excessive cleaning of the ears. Infectious agents such as bacteria and yeast are the most common perpetuating factors of otitis externa (Figure 4.4). They are present in low numbers in normal ears (Tater et al. 2003). These organisms do not cause a problem unless the microenvironment of the ear has been changed by a

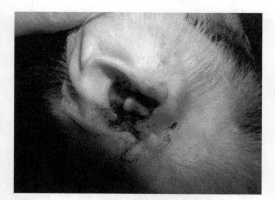

Figure 4.2 Otodectic acariasis; note dark, coffee-ground appearance of discharge. *Source:* Photo by Dr. Sheila Torres, courtesy of the University of Minnesota, College of Veterinary Medicine.

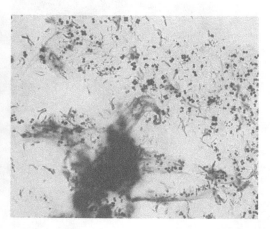

Figure 4.4 Ear cytology (100×) showing cocci and rod bacteria.

predisposing or primary factor that allows them to overgrow. Gram-positive cocci such as *Staphylococcus* spp. and fungal organisms such as *Malassezia pachydermatis* are usually associated with acute otitis externa, while gram-negative bacteria such as *Pseudomonas aeruginosa* are more commonly seen with chronic otitis externa. If otitis externa is not treated and is allowed to progress, otitis media and chronic pathological changes will follow.

Otitis media usually results from inflammation and microbial infection in the external ear canal that extends into the middle ear cavity. Tympanic membrane rupture is common in chronic otitis externa, and this allows purulent exudate and debris to accumulate in the middle ear cavity. Tympanic membranes have a tendency to heal quickly even in the face of active infection. The debris is then trapped in the middle ear cavity and acts as a nidus for reinfection once the external ear canal has been cleared.

The longer the inflammation is left untreated, the more pathological changes may occur in the ear canal wall. The ceruminous glands will start to hypertrophy and cause little visible bumps on the pinna and in the canal. This is sometimes referred to as cobblestone change (Figure 4.5). The epidermis and dermis of the ear canal also start to thicken and fold so that the canal lumen narrows. If the inflammation is not controlled, the external ear canal can close up completely and calcify (Figure 4.6). If this occurs, surgical removal of the external ear canal may be the only option. Fortunately, the ear is fairly forgiving and these changes can at least partially be reversed with treatment and by controlling the underlying predisposing and primary causes of otitis externa.

Contact allergic or irritant reactions to ear medications are a common iatrogenic perpetuating factor of otitis externa (Figure 4.7). Any ingredient in any preparation can cause a problem, including various antibiotics, antifungal agents, and vehicles such as propylene glycol, which is present in many ear medications (Miller et al. 2013). The clinical signs of a contact reaction (erythema,

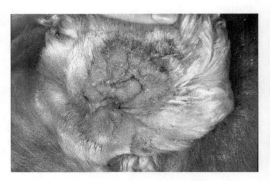

Figure 4.6 End-stage proliferative otitis externa in a cocker spaniel.

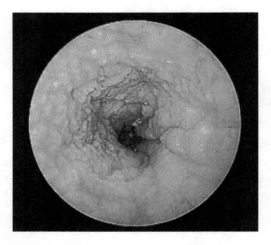

Figure 4.5 Video-otoscopic picture of severe "cobblestone change" in horizontal canal.

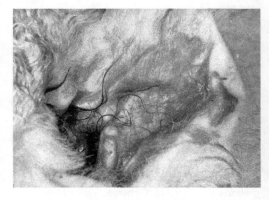

Figure 4.7 Contact reaction to ear medication; note erythema and ulceration of pinnal surface.

ulceration, moist exudate, pain) can be indistinguishable from those of otitis externa. Worsening of clinical signs despite treatment or increased discomfort or pain after application of the ear medication should increase suspicion of a possible contact reaction and the patient should be re-examined quickly.

Clinical Features

Patients with otitis externa can present with similar clinical signs no matter what the underlying primary cause of the otitis. These signs can include erythema of the external ear canal and ear pinna, ceruminous (waxy) or purulent exudate from the ear, erosion or ulceration of the external ear canal, swelling of the external ear canal, foul odor from the ear, pain or pruritus of the ear, head shaking, and a head tilt (Figures 4.8–4.10).

Since otitis externa has a variety of causes, a complete dermatological history and examination are necessary to differentiate between the various predisposing, primary, and perpetuating factors (see Chapter 1 for examples of dermatology history questionnaires). Important questions to ask are whether the otitis is unilateral or bilateral; whether the otitis is a recurrent problem and if so, how old the patient was when the otitis first began; how long the otitis has been present; whether the otitis is a seasonal problem; whether the patient swims; whether there are

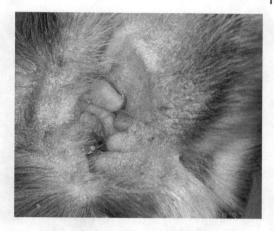

Figure 4.9 Ceruminous exudate of *Malassezia* otitis externa.

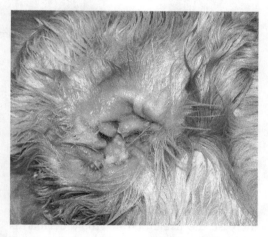

Figure 4.10 Purulent exudate of bacterial otitis externa.

other pets in the household and are they affected; what treatments have been used in the past and what has been the patient's response; whether the client performs routine ear cleaning at home; if the ears are hairy whether the hair is removed routinely; whether the patient has any other skin problems; and whether the patient has any other abnormal clinical signs. Answers to these questions as well as the veterinarian's findings on a complete dermatological exam will provide important clues to the underlying causes of the patient's otitis externa. For example, unilateral otitis externa is more

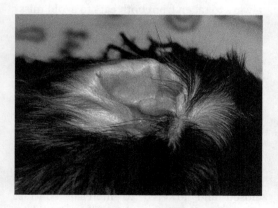

Figure 4.8 Erythematous atopic otitis externa.

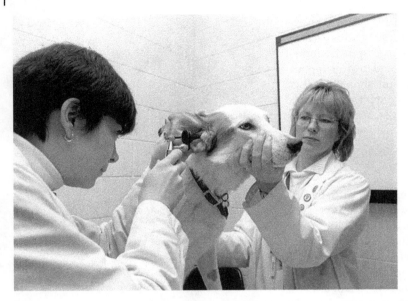

Figure 4.11 Otoscopic exam. *Source:* Photo by Sue Kirchoff, courtesy of the University of Minnesota, College of Veterinary Medicine.

common with foreign bodies or tumors, whereas bilateral otitis externa is more typical for parasitic infestations, allergic skin diseases, and hypothyroidism. Parasitic otitis externa (particularly that caused by *O. cynotis*) is more common in young animals, while tumors are more commonly seen in older patients. Concurrent dermatological signs such as interdigital erythema and pruritus increase the likelihood of atopic dermatitis or food allergy as a potential primary cause of otitis externa.

As part of the complete dermatological exam, the veterinarian will do an otoscopic exam of the ear (Figure 4.11). Ideally, the unaffected or less painful ear should be examined first and a new otoscope cone should be used for each ear. Otoscope cones should be thoroughly cleaned and disinfected after each use, as they can harbor harmful bacteria such as *P. aeruginosa* (Kirby et al. 2010), or you may want to consider using disposable otoscope cones for patients presenting with otitis externa. The otoscope allows visualization of the interior of the vertical and horizontal canals and possibly also the tympanic membrane. If the ears are painful,

swollen, or contain large amounts of exudate at the first visit, a thorough otoscopic exam may not be possible. The ears may need to be treated for several days before an otoscopic examination can be done.

Diagnostic Tests

All cases of otitis externa should have ear swab samples taken to look for parasites, bacteria, and yeast. Even though only one ear may appear to be affected, samples should always to taken from both ears to avoid missing early or very mild cases of otitis externa. To obtain a sample, gently insert the cotton swab into the ear canal to the level of the vertical/horizontal canal junction and rotate to get a good sample of the exudate. Then roll the swab out onto two glass slides, one for cytology and one to look for parasites. The slide for parasite examination should have a drop of mineral oil placed on it and the slide should be examined microscopically under low power (4× and 10×), with the condenser closed and lowered to increase contrast (Figure 4.12). The cytology slide should be

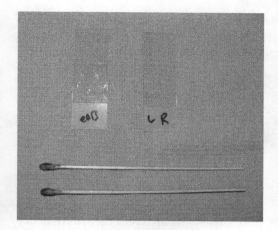

Figure 4.12 Ear cytology slide (slide on right) and ear swab slide with mineral oil for parasite examination (slide on left).

stained with Diff-Quik or new methylene blue and examined under oil immersion with the condenser open and up. The presence of cocci and rod bacteria, *Malassezia* organisms, and inflammatory cells should be noted. Gram staining of cytology slides may also be done.

Bacterial culture and sensitivity testing may be recommended if primarily rod bacteria are seen on cytology. Rods may represent *P. aeruginosa*, *Escherichia coli*, or *Proteus* sp. bacteria, which are generally more difficult to treat. To obtain a sample for bacterial culture, gently insert a sterile swab into the bottom of the vertical canal and rotate to get a good sample of the exudate. Be sure to do this before you use any cleaning agents or flushes in the ear, since these products can adversely affect your culture.

Additional diagnostic testing to investigate primary causes of otitis externa will be based on the patient's history and clinical signs. The veterinarian may recommend a food trial, allergy testing to identify environmental allergens, thyroid hormone level testing, complete blood count and serum biochemistry panel to look for signs of systemic disease, and radiographs or computed tomography (CT) scans to evaluate the middle ear.

Treatment

Treating the patient with otitis externa requires a multi-step approach. The predisposing factors, primary causes, and perpetuating factors of the otic disease must be identified and addressed. Therapy typically includes ear cleaning/flushing, use of antimicrobial agents, and glucocorticoids to decrease otic inflammation. Patients with mild to moderate otitis are generally treated for a three to four week period. A recheck appointment should be scheduled after two to three weeks of treatment. The clinical appearance of the ear along with results of otic cytology will allow the veterinarian to assess the patient's progress. After resolution, some patients may benefit from periodic ear cleaning to prevent recurrence of otitis externa.

Predisposing Factors

Most ear canal anatomical and micro-anatomical variations that predispose dogs to otitis externa are breed related. For this reason, it is important to teach clients preventative ear care when these breeds are puppies. For dogs with pendulous ears, the clients should aerate the ears several times weekly. This means flipping the ear pinnae up onto the head so air can get into the ear canals. They should also use a gentle drying agent once weekly to every other week, especially after bathing and swimming, to dehumidify the canal. In dogs such as spaniels and Labrador retrievers who have more ceruminous glands than other breeds, the owners may need to clean out the ears weekly, since these breeds produce more wax. In some cases because of copious wax production a ceruminolytic (wax remover) and a stronger drying agent are needed.

In poodles or other breeds with hairy ear canals, the client must learn how to properly clean the ears and only remove the hair if and when necessary. These dogs should have their ears cleaned out with a ceruminolytic and a drying agent every one to two weeks. Hair removal is best accomplished using hemostats to extract the hair or gentle chemical depilatories to dissolve the hair. This is best done at the veterinary office. It is important that no powders be used to facilitate hair extraction, since powders can cause a foreign body reaction which can lead to otitis externa. An anti-inflammatory medication should be applied to the ears after the hair is removed to decrease inflammation.

If a dog lives in a humid, warm climate, the owners should use a drying agent weekly to every other week depending on the time of year. This is also true for dogs that are bathed frequently or swim.

Primary Causes

Therapy for primary causes of otitis externa varies with each patient. Parasites are treated with the appropriate parasiticidal agent. Foreign bodies and tumors must be removed from the ear canal. The foreign body may be obvious, or may be hidden in debris and exudate and may be flushed out when a thorough ear cleaning is performed. Some ear masses can be removed with a fiber optic otoscope and laser (usually done by a veterinary dermatologist) and other masses may require surgical removal of part or all of the external ear canal. These cases are typically referred to a boarded surgeon. If the primary cause is allergic dermatitis, management of the underlying allergy is key to preventing relapses of otitis externa.

Perpetuating Factors

Most cases of otitis externa, no matter what the underlying primary cause, present with active infections which must be dealt with immediately. Many may also have otitis media and chronic pathological changes in the canal that must be treated if the otitis externa is to resolve completely. The severity and extent of the microbial infection will determine if topical therapy alone will be adequate or if systemic therapy will also be

needed. If infection is severe, pain medications including non-steroidal anti-inflammatory agents, corticosteroids, or opiates may be needed. Most ear preparations contain an antibiotic, an antifungal agent, and a corticosteroid. Various formulations are available, including solutions, suspensions, creams, and ointments. Ear medications vary in their ease of application and it can sometimes be helpful to use a tuberculin syringe to apply a pre-measured amount of the preparation to the ear rather than counting drops. Medication choice will be determined by the microorganisms involved, the nature of the exudate present, and the severity of the infection. The presence or absence of the tympanic membrane should also be considered when choosing ear medications, since some antimicrobials are potentially ototoxic.

Ear Cleaning

The most important first step in the management of any case of otitis is proper cleaning of the external ear canal. Ideally, the initial cleaning is done in the veterinary clinic. This ensures a clean ear at the start of treatment and also allows demonstration of the correct cleaning technique for the client. In mild cases of otitis, ear flushing may be done with gentle restraint. In most cases the ears are painful enough to warrant at least heavy sedation. In more severe cases of otitis externa, especially if otitis media is present, general anesthesia with endotracheal intubation is necessary. Intubation and inflation of the endotracheal tube cuff protect the lower airways from accidental introduction of pathogenic organisms from the middle ear via the Eustachian tube. If the canals are extremely inflamed and swollen, therapy that includes systemic and topical glucocorticoids should be initiated and the ear cleaning should be postponed. This allows the tissue in the canal to become less swollen and friable, so the debris can be removed and the tympanic membrane can be more easily visualized. The flushing solution used depends on the degree of inflammation, the characteristics of the discharge, and the status of the tympanic membrane.

A wide variety of ear cleansers are available, ranging from strong ceruminolytics that must be thoroughly rinsed out of the ear (or they will cause inflammation) to leave-in mild cleansers and drying agents. Many of these cleansers also have antiseptic properties. All ear cleaning solutions except saline and squalene have the potential to damage exposed middle ear structures (Mansfield et al. 1997), although the caseous or purulent material being removed poses just as great if not a greater threat to the delicate structures of the middle ear if left there. When the tympanum is known to be absent, a gentle solution such as warm or room-temperature water or saline should be employed if possible. Unfortunately, many times these solutions alone will not remove the debris and a stronger cleaning solution must be used. At the end of the procedure it is important to completely flush the cleaning solution out of the external canal and middle ear cavity with water or saline.

Ear cleaning in the veterinary office can be as simple as filling the ear canals with the flushing solution, gently massaging the base of the ear, and wiping out the discharge with cotton balls. This procedure may be sufficient for mild otitis externa with minimal exudate. For cases with more exudate in the ears, flushing with a bulb syringe is a good option and can be done with the patient awake or sedated (Figure 4.13). The ear canals should be filled with the cleaning solution and allowed to soak for 5–10 minutes. Then fill the bulb syringe with warm water or saline, insert the tip into the opening of the ear canal, and flush the exudate and debris out of the canal (Figure 4.14). Be sure to allow room around the bulb syringe tip for material

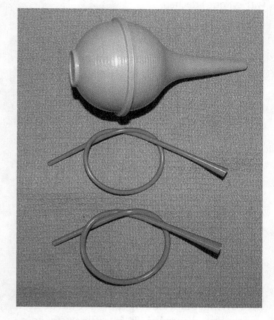

Figure 4.13 Bulb syringe and red rubber feeding tubes.

(a)

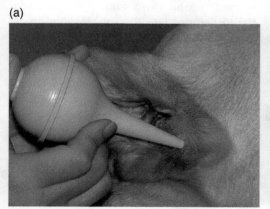

(b)

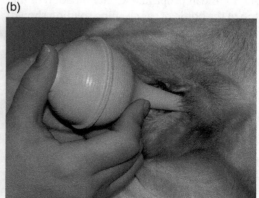

Figure 4.14 (a and b) Bulb syringe placement in ear canal.

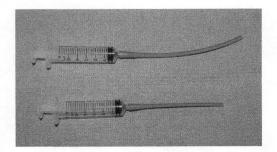

Figure 4.15 Red rubber feeding tubes, trimmed with syringe attached.

to flow out of the ear canal. Continue flushing until no more exudate and debris is visible. Then follow with application of a small amount of cleanser that is safe to leave in the ear, or the first dose of ear medication.

With patients under general anesthesia, the proximal horizontal canal and the middle ear cavity can be flushed with red rubber feeding tubes and warm saline or water. The red rubber tube should be cut to approximately 1.5–2 times the length of the external ear canal and the open end will need to be trimmed to accommodate the tip of a syringe (Figure 4.15). Tom cat catheters or other more rigid tubing are not recommended for ear flushing, since it is much easier to puncture healthy ear drums with these products. Bulb syringes and feeding tubes should be used once, then discarded. It is difficult to completely sterilize the rubber; therefore, resistant strains of *P. aeruginosa*, *E. coli*, and *Proteus mirabilis* can propagate. Contamination of the top of the bottle of ear cleaning solution should also be avoided.

It is very important to be gentle when flushing both cat and dog ears. This is particularly true for cats, as they experience complications from ear cleanings at a higher rate than dogs. Be sure not to pull too hard on the pinnae and not to insert the bulb syringe too deep into the canal so that a seal is formed that does not allow excess liquid to drain out of the ear. Also be sure to always massage the base of the ear canal gently. Excessively vigorous massage can rupture the tympanic membrane. Once the horizontal

canal has been cleaned, it is usually easier for the veterinarian to assess the status of the tympanic membrane.

The hazards of deep ear cleaning include inadvertent rupture of the tympanic membrane, Horner's syndrome, vestibular dysfunction, auditory dysfunction, contact irritant/allergy, and introduction of other pathogens. The most common complication that occurs is rupture of the tympanic membrane. A normal tympanum is difficult to rupture; therefore, if the membrane ruptures with gentle manipulation it was probably weakened and diseased. The occurrence of vestibular or auditory dysfunction is unpredictable. In the dog it is uncommon, usually mild, and most of the time lasts only a few hours to a couple of days. In the cat it occurs more frequently than in the dog and the signs are usually more pronounced and may be permanent. To avoid contact irritation, a gentle solution should be used whenever possible or stronger cleaning solutions must be rinsed out extremely well with warm water or saline. New pathogens can be introduced into an already inflamed ear with unsterilized ear cleaning equipment or contaminated products.

Once the ear has been cleaned in the office, a flushing plan for the client to do at home must be designed. Factors to consider include the organism(s) found on cytology or culture, the severity of the ear disease, the type and amount of exudate produced, and the status of the tympanic membrane. It is also essential to demonstrate the ear cleaning procedure to the client (see Chapter 1 for helpful hints with ear cleaning). The client will need to know how much solution to use, how to apply it, what can be safely used to wipe the debris out of the ears, and how deep into the canal it is safe to go. For most cases a prepared solution in a squeeze bottle is all that is necessary. If there is a great deal of purulent discharge, flushing with a bulb syringe might be needed. If a bulb syringe is to be used more than once, it should be rinsed out several times with a 50/50 white vinegar/alcohol mixture to minimize bacterial growth in the bulb. The bulb syringe should be changed frequently.

It is important to remember that purulent discharge will inactivate many topical antibiotics, so the ear should be flushed prior to each application of antibiotic until the ear is producing little to no purulent material. Initially, the frequency of flushing for severe cases may be once to twice daily. As therapy continues, the frequency should decrease to several times a week, then once weekly to every other week.

It is particularly important that dogs with chronic pathological ear canal changes such as fibrosis, stenosis, and lichenification be placed on a maintenance flushing program. Ears with chronic changes usually have increased cerumen production, increased stratum corneum production, and decreased epidermal migration. This leads to an increased buildup of debris in the canal. Flushing the ears helps to remove the debris and acidify the canal. This assists in preventing the recurrence of active infections. The frequency of flushing ranges from two to three times weekly to once every other week. Although flushing is extremely important in the management of both chronic and acute otitis, it is imperative to remember that flushing too vigorously and too frequently can also be detrimental to the otic epidermis. The patient with severe otitis whose ears are being flushed frequently should be checked often and flushing varied depending on cytology and otic examination. This will prevent damage to the ear canal epithelium from excessive flushing.

Client Education

Helping clients understand the complex nature of otitis externa is crucial to achieving good compliance with treatment recommendations. What to them looks like a simple "ear infection" is the result of a combination of predisposing factors, primary causes, and perpetuating factors of otitis externa. It is helpful to explain to the client that there is an underlying cause for the microbial infection and that treating the secondary infection is only part of the therapy. Although recurrent ear infections may look the same to the client, they need to understand that an exam and cytology are always necessary to determine the microbe(s) involved so that the appropriate therapy can be prescribed. Predisposing factors must also be addressed and identifying the underlying primary cause of the otitis is important for preventing recurrence of otitis externa.

The technician should show the client how to clean the ears and how to apply the ear medication. Demonstrating how much solution to apply, how long to let it soak, how to gently massage the base of the ear, and how to wipe out the exudate and cleaning solution are all important steps of the process. Clients should be shown how to apply cleaner and medication without contaminating the containers and without transferring exudate and microorganisms from one ear to the other. It can be a valuable exercise to treat one ear and then have the client treat the other ear to ensure they have learned the correct procedure and feel comfortable performing this at home. If clients are having difficulties with at home flushing, giving them the option to have the flushing performed at the veterinary clinic, as a technician appointment is an added service that can improve compliance. Each client should go home with a set of written instructions that details how often the ears are to be cleaned and medicated, and, ideally, a handout describing the ear cleaning procedure.

The importance of keeping recheck appointments must also be stressed. Repeat otoscopic exams and ear cytology are used to evaluate response to treatment and to determine when treatment can stop and when the frequency of cleaning can decrease. The external ear canal opening may look normal before the deeper parts of the ear canal have cleared. Stopping treatment before the otitis externa has resolved completely will guarantee a recurrence of the problem. It is also important to make clients aware of the possibility of ototoxic reactions and contact reactions. The owner should be warned to watch for hearing loss or dizziness, which may indicate an ototoxic reaction. Also they should watch for any worsening of the redness, pain, or discharge, since these may indicate a contact reaction. If they notice any of these changes they should stop the medications and call the office immediately.

Conclusion

Otitis externa can be a frustrating condition for many clients. The technician can help prevent some of this frustration by making sure the client understands that there is more to otitis externa than the obvious microbial infection. Recognizing and controlling the underlying causes of the infection are key to preventing recurrent otitis externa. The technician's role is also essential in the education of the client on how to properly flush and medicate the ears. Finally, the technician can help ensure that the client continues maintenance therapies by communicating with them on a regular basis. Good client communication will go a long way toward successful management of otitis externa cases.

References

Bensignor, E. and Forsythe, P.J. (2012). An approach to otitis externa. In: *BSAVA Manual of Canine and Feline Dermatology*, 3e (eds. H.A. Jackson and R. Marsella), 110–120. Gloucester UK: British Small Animal Veterinary Association.

Kirby, A.L., Rosenkrantz, W.S., Ghubash, R.M. et al. (2010). Evaluation of otoscope cone disinfection techniques and contamination level in small animal private practice. *Veterinary Dermatology* 21 (2): 175–183.

Mansfield, P.D., Steiss, J.E., Boosinger, T.R., and Marshall, A.E. (1997). The effects of four commercial ceruminolytic agents on the middle ear. *Journal of American Animal Hospital Association* 33 (6): 479–486.

Miller, W.H., Griffin, C.E., and Campbell, K.L. (2013). *Muller & Kirk's Small Animal Dermatology*, 7e. St. Louis, MO: Elsevier/ Mosby.

Nationwide (2018). Most common medical conditions that prompt veterinary visits. https://press8.petinsurance.com/ articles/2018/march/most-common-medical-conditions-that-prompt-veterinary-visits (accessed May 2019).

Tater, K.C., Scott, D.W., Miller, W.H., and Erb, H.N. (2003). The cytology of the external ear in the normal dog and cat. *Journal of Veterinary Medicine. Series B* 50 (7): 370–374.

5

Dermatophytosis
Sandra Grable

Introduction

Dermatophytosis is a relatively uncommon condition seen in clinical practice (Miller et al. 2013a, Moriello and DeBoer 2012); however, prompt recognition and treatment of dermatophytosis are critical due to the contagious and zoonotic nature of this disease. Successful management of these cases can be challenging and requires extensive client education. Recognizing clinical signs during the physical examination, preparing and evaluating fungal cultures, minimizing contagion for hospital staff, and preventing contamination in the clinic as well as the home are just a few of the veterinary technician's responsibilities. Managing dermatophytosis in animal shelters or catteries becomes even more challenging, and the reader is encouraged to obtain more information on this subject from the recommended reading listed at the end of the chapter.

Pathogenesis

Dermatophytosis is a contagious and zoonotic, superficial fungal skin disease commonly referred to as "ringworm." It received this designation due to the appearance of the classic circular, scaling lesions often produced in humans. Dermatophytic fungi obtain their nutrients from digestion of keratin, a protein found in the hair, superficial epidermis (stratum corneum), and claws. Transmission occurs when there is direct contact with infected hairs or skin scales on other animals or humans, in the environment, or on fomites such as bedding, crates, brushes, and other grooming equipment. Fungal spores within infected hairs can remain viable for up to 18 months and can be a significant source for reinfection (Miller et al. 2013a; Moriello and DeBoer 2012). The typical incubation period is one to three weeks; however, exposure does not always lead to infection. The degree of exposure, damage to the skin's barrier function, and host immunocompetency all affect the likelihood of infection (Moriello and DeBoer 2012). Normal cat grooming behavior may remove fungal spores and help prevent infection. Dermatophytosis is usually a self-limiting disease in healthy animals, with most cases resolving in two to three months. Treatment is still recommended due to the contagious and zoonotic nature of this disease (Moriello and DeBoer 2012).

The three dermatophytes that most commonly infect dogs and cats are *Microsporum canis*, *Microsporum gypseum*, and *Trichophyton mentagrophytes*. *M. canis* causes the vast majority of dermatophytosis in cats, while dogs are affected by all three species (Moriello and DeBoer 2014). These fungi are not normal inhabitants of feline or canine haircoats and isolation of a dermatophyte from an

Small Animal Dermatology for Technicians and Nurses, First Edition. Edited by Kim Horne, Marcia Schwassmann and Dawn Logas.
© 2020 John Wiley & Sons, Inc. Published 2020 by John Wiley & Sons, Inc.

asymptomatic animal indicates either very early infection or temporary fomite status (Moriello and DeBoer 2012). Dermatophytes are classified as geophilic (from the soil), anthropophilic (from humans), or zoophilic (from animals). Cats are often the source of *M. canis* infections, *M. gypseum* is typically acquired from the soil, and rodents are often the source of *T. mentagrophytes* infections (Miller et al. 2013a).

Clinical Features

Obtaining an accurate and in-depth patient history is an important aspect of any dermatological examination. There are particular questions to ask clients when dermatophytosis is suspected. Since dermatophytosis is contagious as well as zoonotic, it is important to know if any other pets or humans in the household are affected. The age of the patient is also relevant, since younger and older animals may be more susceptible to infection (Miller et al. 2013a). Immunosuppression due to concurrent illness (e.g. feline leukemia virus or feline immunodeficiency virus infection) or immunosuppressive drug therapy can also predispose to dermatophytosis (Miller et al. 2013a). Breed predilections have been reported with Yorkshire terriers, Manchester terriers, and long-haired cats, such as Persians, being more susceptible to dermatophytosis (Miller et al. 2013a).

Environmental questions are also very important: Does the pet spend any time outdoors? Does it come in contact with wildlife, root around in soil, or stick its nose in rodent holes? Does the pet go to the groomer, daycare facilities, dog or cat shows, or dog parks? Does it attend obedience or conformation classes? Does the owner care for stray dogs or cats? Does the pet ever go to a boarding kennel? These pets with potential for contact with numerous animals are at higher risk for dermatophytosis.

Dermatophytosis causes varying degrees of pruritus, ranging from none to severe (Miller et al. 2013a; Moriello and DeBoer 2012).

Owners should be asked about their pet's degree of itchiness, being careful to include licking, biting, and chewing as well as scratching as indicators of pruritus.

Clinical signs of dermatophytosis are highly variable (Figures 5.1 and 5.2). Single to multiple patches of alopecia, with varying degrees of erythema and crusting, are the most common presentation of dermatophytosis in dogs and cats. Dogs can also present with follicular papules and pustules. Circular areas of alopecia with a peripheral crust and central area of healing (epidermal collarettes) can be seen with dermatophytosis, but more often indicate the presence of bacterial folliculitis in dogs. Severe cases can present with extensive alopecia, crusting, hyperpigmentation, and furuncles. Nodular lesions called kerions (Figures 5.3 and 5.4) are seen more

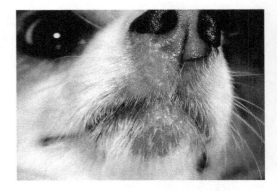

Figure 5.1 Facial lesions cultured positive for *Trichophyton mentagrophytes*.

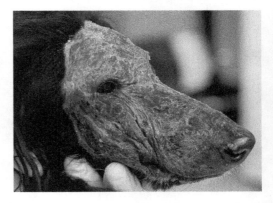

Figure 5.2 Severe *Trichophyton* infection on a dog.

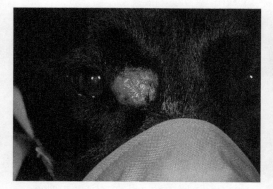

Figure 5.3 Fungal kerion cultured positive for *Trichophyton mentagrophytes*.

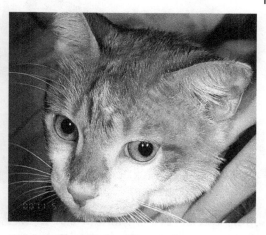

Figure 5.5 Erythema and alopecia from *Microsporum canis* infection.

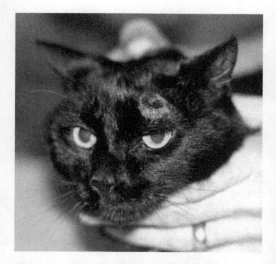

Figure 5.4 Fungal kerion diagnosed via biopsy. *Source:* Courtesy of Dawn Logas DVM, DACVD.

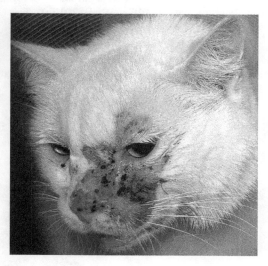

Figure 5.6 Facial erythema, alopecia, crusting, and excoriations from pruritic *Microsporum canis* infection. *Source:* Courtesy of Dawn Logas DVM, DACVD.

often with *M. gypseum* and *T. mentagrophytes* infections. Onychomycosis (fungal infection of the nails) is uncommon and is usually associated with *T. mentagrophytes* infection (Miller et al. 2013a). Nails on one or more feet can be affected and may be misshapen, soft, crumbly, or brittle. The nail folds and feet may also show signs of dermatophytosis.

Cats have an even wider variety of presentations of dermatophytosis (Figures 5.5–5.7). Clinical signs can vary from barely visible inflammation or alopecia on the face or ear pinnae to large patches of alopecia with

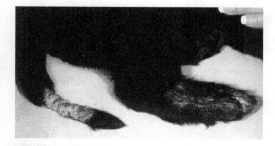

Figure 5.7 *Microsporum gypseum* infection in a cat. *Source:* Courtesy of Dawn Logas, DVM, DACVD.

varying degrees of erythema and scaling. Cats with very subtle lesions easily missed on physical examination were previously labeled as asymptomatic carriers. These patients probably have either very early clinical disease or are acting as temporary fomites (Moriello 2016). Miliary dermatitis (multiple crusted papules), lesions of chin acne (papules, alopecia, comedones, furuncles, draining tracts, and crusting), hyperpigmentation, paronychia, excessive shedding, eosinophilic plaques, and indolent ulcers have all been associated with feline dermatophytosis (Miller et al. 2013a; Moriello and DeBoer 2012). Cats do not usually develop kerions, but pseudomycetomas, subcutaneous nodules that may ulcerate and drain can be seen in Persian cats (Miller et al. 2013a). The lesions produced by dermatophytosis can also be seen with bacterial folliculitis, demodicosis, or even auto-immune diseases such as pemphigus foliaceus (Peters et al. 2007). Therefore, dermatophytosis cannot be diagnosed based on clinical signs alone.

Diagnostic Tests

The great variability of clinical signs seen with dermatophytosis makes diagnostic testing crucial for accurate identification of this disease.

Woods Lamp Examination

Examination of hairs with a Wood's lamp (ultraviolet light source) can be a useful screening tool for diagnosing dermatophytosis. Some strains of *M. canis* produce fungal metabolites that cause infected hairs to show apple-green fluorescence when exposed to light from a Wood's lamp (Figures 5.8 and 5.9). Plug-in versions of Wood's lamps are preferred over battery-operated ones and the lamp should be allowed to warm up for several minutes before use, since its light intensity and stability are temperature dependent (Moriello and DeBoer 2012). It is

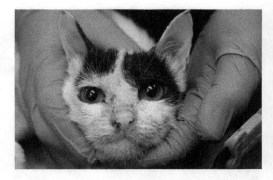

Figure 5.8 Facial crusts and alopecia on a feline patient with *Microsporum canis*. *Source:* Courtesy of Amelia G. White, DVM, MS, DACVD, Auburn University, Auburn, AL.

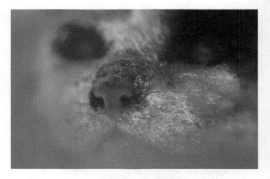

Figure 5.9 Fluorescing hairs on a feline patient using the Wood's lamp. *Source:* Courtesy of Amelia G. White, DVM, MS, DACVD, Auburn University, Auburn, AL.

necessary to turn off the room lights to allow your eyes to adjust to the darkness and to see the fluorescence. The patient's entire haircoat should be carefully examined for fluorescent hairs. Wood's lamp examination cannot rule out dermatophytosis, since only about half the strains of *M. canis* fluoresce (Moriello and DeBoer 2012). False positive results are also common. Carpet fibers, lint, debris, topical medications, and crusts often fluoresce upon Wood's lamp examination, so it is important to distinguish this fluorescence from the apple-green fluorescence of hair shafts that indicates possible dermatophytosis. If fluorescing hairs are identified, these hairs should be selected for direct examination and fungal culture.

Trichography

Direct microscopic examination (trichography) of hairs can be used to identify fungal spores (arthroconidia) along the outside of the hair shaft, an ectothrix distribution, and fungal hyphae within the hair shaft. Although it is an inexpensive test that can be completed during the appointment, trichography does require considerable expertise on the part of the veterinarian or technician performing the examination. If this test is positive, it is considered diagnostic for dermatophytosis and treatment can be initiated while waiting for fungal culture results to identify the species of dermatophyte involved. A negative result on direct examination of hairs does not, however, rule out dermatophytosis.

To perform trichography, pluck hairs in the direction they grow from the periphery of suspicious lesions, scrape suspicious lesions, or select hairs that fluoresced on Wood's lamp examination (Moriello and DeBoer 2012). Place the hairs and scraped material on a glass slide with mineral oil, add a coverslip, and examine the hair shafts. View the slide starting with a low power objective and work up, using care with the higher objectives as mineral oil can damage the 40× objective. The condenser on the microscope should be lowered to increase contrast for easier identification of spores or hyphae. Look for damaged hair shafts to examine. Infected hairs may have a swollen or frayed appearance. Fungal hyphae may be seen within the hair shafts and chains of conidia may be seen surrounding the hairs (Figure 5.10).

It is important to remember that dermatophytes never produce macroconidia when growing in tissue, only when growing on culture media. Therefore, any macroconidia present represent environmental contamination with saprophytic fungi (Miller et al. 2013b; Moriello and DeBoer 2012). Practice is required to become proficient in this technique. It is best to start by examining hairs from known positive animals. Remember that a negative result on trichography does not rule out the diagnosis of dermatophytosis.

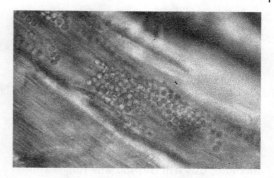

Figure 5.10 Direct microscopic examination of a hair showing ectothrix spores (40×).

Fungal Culture

Fungal culture is the most reliable and widely used method for diagnosis of dermatophytosis. Hairs, scale, and crusts should be collected using similar techniques as described for trichography. Samples should be taken from the periphery of lesions, since this is where the actively growing fungal organisms are most likely to be found. Use hemostats to pull suspicious-looking hairs out at their base close to the skin. Cut off and discard the tips of long hairs. This allows hairs to fit better onto the fungal culture plate and reduces contamination of the culture with saprophytic fungi. Take samples from several different areas of the lesion and take samples from different locations if multiple lesions are present. To decrease the degree of culture contamination with saprophytic fungi, you can gently wipe the area to be cultured with 70% isopropyl alcohol and let it air dry before collecting samples (Miller et al. 2013b; Moriello and DeBoer 2012).

The Mackenzie toothbrush collection technique is another way to collect samples for culturing. This method is especially useful for identifying asymptomatic carriers or when treated animals are returning for follow-up cultures when they are no longer exhibiting obvious lesions. A new toothbrush is used to repeatedly brush suspicious lesions, or the entire animal if no lesions are present. This process should take two to three minutes (Moriello and DeBoer 2012). A new toothbrush in its original packaging should be free of dermatophytes and does not need to be sterilized prior to use (Moriello and DeBoer 2012). Be sure to brush the face and inside of the ear pinnae in cats, since these are common areas for early lesions of dermatophytosis (Moriello and DeBoer 2012). After collecting hair and scale samples, repeatedly and gently touch the bristles of the toothbrush directly onto the culture medium; this will transfer any fungal spores onto the surface of the medium. In addition, you may also pull the hairs from the bristles and place them onto the medium using hemostats. Inexpensive toothbrushes with bristles in an even, horizontal plane collect hairs most efficiently and can be bought in bulk and disposed of properly after a single use. Owners with multiple-pet households can use this technique to collect samples at home. Toothbrushes can be placed in individual plastic bags or envelopes labeled with each patient's name. This eliminates the need to bring multiple infected animals to the clinic and reduces environmental contamination of the owner's vehicle and the veterinary hospital (Moriello and DeBoer 2012).

When onychomycosis is suspected, the area around the claw and the claw itself should be cleansed with 70% alcohol and allowed to air dry before samples are obtained (Miller et al. 2013b). A #10 scalpel blade can be used to gently scrape the concave surface of the claw as far back or proximal as possible (Moriello and DeBoer 2012). Hair samples from near the nails should also be collected. Place the material collected onto the fungal medium by pressing it lightly onto the surface. The Mackenzie brush technique can also be used to collect samples from around the nail (Moriello and DeBoer 2012). If brittle or detached nails are present, they may be clipped and also placed on the culture medium.

Fungal cultures of samples from the surface of nodular lesions such as kerions are often negative. Fungal hyphae or arthroconidia may be seen on cytology of exudate or fine needle aspirate from these lesions (Cornegliani et al. 2009; Logan et al. 2006).

Once samples have been collected, inoculate the culture plate by gently placing the hairs and scale on top of the dermatophyte test medium (DTM). Lay the hairs flat ensuring good contact with the medium, since it contains the nutrients the dermatophytes need to grow. A common mistake is to place a large amount of hair in a clump on top of the medium with most hairs actually in free space, and only a few in contact with the medium. One should also avoid embedding the hairs deeply into the medium, since dermatophytes are aerobic organisms.

Although this chapter is limited to dogs and cats, it is worth mentioning that DTM should not be used for culturing dermatophytes from large animals. Some of the dermatophyte species that infect large animals have different nutritional requirements that are not met by DTM (Scott and Miller 2003).

It has long been thought that light inhibits growth of dermatophytes, but a recent publication suggests this may not be true (Verbrugge et al. 2008). If an incubator is available, this is ideal, since the temperature and light can be controlled more consistently. If needed, a small container of tap water can be placed in the incubator along with the cultures to keep them from drying out. If an incubator is not available, keep the cultures away from heating and air-conditioning vents/ducts and store them at a temperature between 25 and 30 °C (77–86 °F; Verbrugge et al. 2008); anything cooler may slow colony growth and sporulation. Room temperature in many clinics will be substantially lower than the ideal incubation temperature of 25–30 °C (77–86 °F). Most dermatophytes will grow within 14 days, but fungal cultures should be kept for a minimum of 21 days, especially if cultures are from patients on treatment (Moriello and DeBoer 2012). Dermatophyte growth on these culture plates may take longer to appear.

Once the DTM has been inoculated, it should be labeled with the date the culture was started, the patient's and client's names, and the medical record number if applicable. Culture plates should be examined every one to two days and observations should be recorded in a log book (see Table 5.1). For each entry note the date, presence or absence of fungal growth, colony color (both top and underside of colony), any color change of the medium, and microscopic examination findings if applicable. Record the final result in the patient's medical record and notify the veterinarian of any positive or suspicious findings as soon as they appear.

Fungal Culture Media and Systems

DTM is the standard medium used for culturing dermatophytes. It is Sabouraud dextrose agar with cycloheximide, gentamicin, chlortetracycline, and phenol red added. Cycloheximide is an antifungal agent that inhibits the growth of saprophytic fungi, gentamicin and chlortetracycline are antibiotics that inhibit bacterial growth on the medium, and phenol red is a pH indicator (Miller et al. 2013b). Dermatophytes digest protein in the medium first, producing alkaline metabolites that cause phenol red to turn the DTM from yellow to red. After the dermatophytes have exhausted the protein in the DTM, they will use the carbohydrate in the medium. This produces acid metabolites that cause the phenol red to change the DTM from red back to yellow. Most saprophytic fungi use carbohydrates in the DTM first, so will not produce an initial color change of the medium from yellow to red.

There are several culture systems on the market to choose from. The author prefers a dual-plate system with DTM on one side and plain Sabouraud dextrose agar on the other side. The absence of a pH indicator in the plain Sabouraud agar makes visualization of the color of the underside of the dermatophyte colony easier. Some clinicians prefer a combination of DTM on one side of the plate and either rapid sporulation medium (RSM) or enhanced sporulation agar (ESA) on the other side. RSM and ESA are designed to promote the formation of macroconidia. The author does not recommend the small jars filled halfway with DTM on a slant for the following reasons: it is impossible to fit a toothbrush into some jars if the Mackenzie brush technique has been used to collect samples; the surface area of DTM available for dermatophyte growth is relatively small; and a sample of the colony cannot be easily obtained for the microscopic examination of macroconidia that allows identification of the dermatophyte species present.

DTM is also available in a small tray that is designed to be placed directly onto the microscope stage for viewing of macroconidia. This decreases sample handling by eliminating the need to make slides from samples of the colony growth. This tray system is also not recommended, however, due to the small size of the individual squares of DTM. Saprophytes can easily overgrow and obscure a dermatophyte colony on the small square, and the fungal mycelial growth can be too thick to allow visualization of the macroconidia.

Gross Analysis and Microscopy

Dermatophyte colonies will be lightly pigmented, white to cream to beige in color, and will have a cottony, wooly, or powdery texture. Dermatophyte colonies are never darkly pigmented, for instance dark green, dark brown, or black. The color of the underside of a dermatophyte colony can also be evaluated if grown on medium that does not contain a pH indicator. The underside of a dermatophyte colony may be yellow, yellow-orange, tan, red, or brown (Moriello and DeBoer 2012). Dermatophyte colony growth should be accompanied by a color change from yellow to red of the DTM. This is due to the dermatophyte's preference for protein in the DTM as a food source. Protein metabolism produces acid metabolites that cause the pH indicator to turn red. Saprophytes will utilize the carbohydrate in the DTM first and protein second, so the DTM will eventually turn red, but only when the fungal colony is older. This delayed color change is why daily to every other day examination of fungal cultures is necessary.

Any suspicious colonies should be examined microscopically to identify the species

Table 5.1 Example of a log to record culture and microscopic observations/results.

Date/culture age Keep track of culture from day of inoculation and make observations and record for a minimum of 21 days	Medical record number and/or patient name	Client's last name	Observations	Veterinarian notified	Owner notified	Results recorded in medical record	Final results
27 Oct 16/Inoculation	Zeus	Smith					
28 Oct 16/1	Zeus	Smith	No growth				
31 Oct 16/4	Zeus	Smith	No growth				
2 Nov 16/6	Zeus	Smith	White colony growth with media color change				
4 Nov 16/8	Zeus	Smith	Tape mount sample: macroconidia – *Microsporum canis*	Dr. Jones via email at 2:00 p.m.	Spoke with Ms. Smith via phone call at 2:30 p.m.	Entered results in computer at 2:06 p.m.	
10 Nov 16/14	Zeus	Smith	Grayish colony growth, no media color change Tape mount sample: *Alternaria* spp.				
17 Nov 16/21	Zeus	Smith	No additional growth or observations. *M. canis* and *Alternaria* spp.	Dr. Jones via email at 9:00 a.m.		Entered results in computer at 4:15 p.m.	*M. canis* and *Alternaria* spp.

of dermatophyte involved. The species of dermatophyte found will help determine the source of infection, and will influence treatment and environmental decontamination recommendations. A few species of saprophytic fungi are capable of producing an immediate red color change on DTM, so all lightly pigmented colonies should be examined microscopically. Rare variants of *M. canis* have been identified that do not produce a red color change on DTM (Moriello and DeBoer 2012). If an aberrant colony is identified, the fungal culture should be sent to a diagnostic laboratory for identification.

Once colony growth is evident, one can begin microscopic examinations. Most colonies will start producing macroconidia after five to seven days of growth. Suspicious colonies should be examined microscopically every two to three days if no macroconidia are found at first.

To sample the colony, gently press the sticky side of a strip of clear acetate tape to the colony surface. Place a drop of fungal stain (lactophenol cotton blue or new methylene blue) on a glass slide and place the tape onto the stain with the sticky side down. The slide can be examined as is or a second drop

of stain can be placed on top of the tape followed by a cover slip. Lactophenol cotton blue and new methylene blue will stain fungal structures a light blue color.

Scan the slide with the low power objective (4× or 10× lens) first to identify the presence of macroconidia. Then switch to the higher power 40× objective to examine the macroconidia in detail. Lowering the condenser will increase contrast and make identification of macroconidia features easier (see Table 5.2).

M. canis colonies are white and cottony on the surface with a yellow-orange underside. They usually produce large numbers of spindle-shaped macroconidia with thick, spiny walls and a knob on the distal end. Six or more cells in the macroconidia are typical, but young macroconidia may have fewer cells (Figures 5.11 and 5.12).

M. gypseum colonies are buff to cinnamon brown and may have a white periphery. The center of the colony can appear slightly raised and has a granular texture with a yellow to tan underside. The ellipsoid macroconidia have thinner walls and no knob on the end. Fewer than six cells are typical (Figures 5.13 and 5.14).

Table 5.2 Typical colony and microscopic morphology of small animal dermatophytes.

ORGANISM	COLONY	MICROSCOPY
Microsporum canis	• Whitish • Wispy to cottony	• 6 or more septa • Spindle-shaped • Thick, spiny walls • Pinched/tapered ends
Microsporum gypseum	• White at first • Tan center with age • Powdery to granular	• Fewer than 6 septa • Ellipsoid • Thin-walled
Trichophyton mentagrophytes	• White, tan, yellow, or pinkish • Powdery, granular, or downy	• 1–6 septa • Cigar-shaped • Thin, smooth walls • Macroconidia *may be absent* • Clustered microconidia • Spiral hyphae

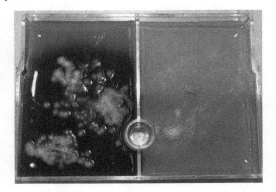

Figure 5.11 *Microsporum canis* colony on dermatophyte test medium (right) and rapid sporulation medium (left).

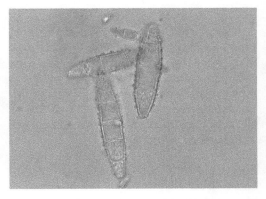

Figure 5.14 Club-shaped macroconidia of *Microsporum gypseum* (40×).

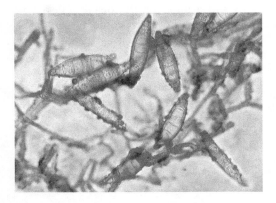

Figure 5.12 *Microsporum canis* macroconidia stained with PMS (40×).

T. mentagrophytes colonies are usually flat and white to cream on the surface. The colony underside can range from tan to brown to red. Cigar-shaped macroconidia with smooth, thin walls are rarely produced. Microconidia are more abundant and spiral hyphae may be noted. These cultures can be sent to a diagnostic laboratory for definitive identification (Figures 5.15–5.17).

Non-pathogenic fungi (saprophytes) are common contaminants on fungal culture plates because their airborne spores are normally present on dog and cat haircoats. Contaminants may be more abundant on plates when the Mackenzie brush technique is used for sample collection. If a contaminant threatens to overgrow a suspected dermatophyte colony, the desired colony can be

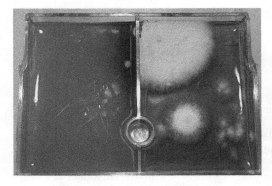

Figure 5.13 *Microsporum gypseum* colony on dermatophyte test medium (right); rapid sporulation medium (left) has no growth. Notice the umbonal, tan center with the larger (older) colony and granular appearance.

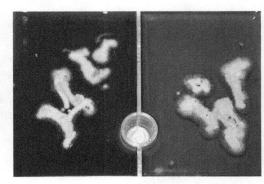

Figure 5.15 *Trichophyton mentagrophytes* colony. Granular appearance and whitish/pink color.

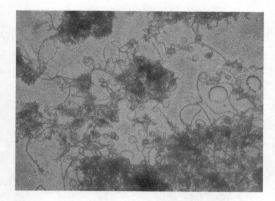

Figure 5.16 Numerous spiral hyphae found on cytology from a *Trichophyton mentagrophytes* colony.

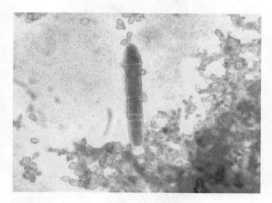

Figure 5.17 Macroconidia of *Trichophyton mentagrophytes*.

rescued by transferring part of it to a new plate using a sterile needle or inoculation loop. Familiarity with the appearance of common contaminants can increase the technician's confidence in identification of the organisms that are pathogenic.

Common Contaminants

Saprophytic fungi often found on fungal cultures include *Alternaria* spp., *Aspergillus* spp., *Cladosporium* spp., *Fusarium* spp., *Penicillium* spp., *Mucor* spp., and *Rhizopus* spp.

Alternaria spp. grow as wooly, whitish-gray colonies that darken as they age. The conidia resemble hand grenades and can have both longitudinal and transverse septae,

unlike dermatophyte macroconidia which only have parallel transverse septae. *Alternaria* spp. conidia may be found singly or in chains (Figure 5.18).

Aspergillus colony color varies depending on the species cultured, ranging from white early on in its growth to shades of green, yellow, red, brown, or black as the colony ages (Larone 2002). Colony texture is velvety or cottony. *Aspergillus* spp. produce conidia that resemble a dandelion gone to seed (Figure 5.19).

Cladosporium spp. produce olive-green to black colonies with a dense, velvety texture. This is one of the few fragile organisms that will not stay intact when performing a tape mount and only bits and pieces of the

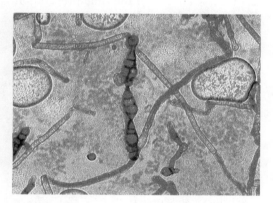

Figure 5.18 *Alternaria* spp. in a chain of three, resembling "hand grenades."

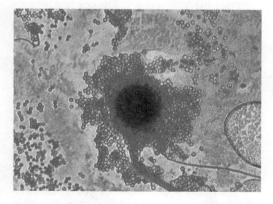

Figure 5.19 *Aspergillus* spp. resembling a "dandelion gone to seed."

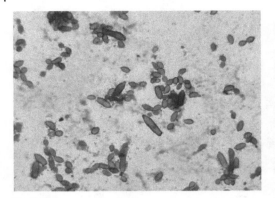

Figure 5.20 Broken conidia from a *Cladosporium* colony.

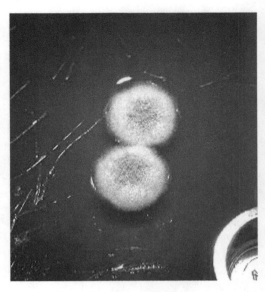

Figure 5.21 Characteristic culture of *Penicillium* spp.

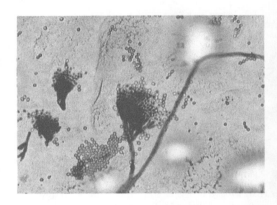

Figure 5.22 *Penicillium* spp. resembling "pitchforks."

organism will be seen, no matter how careful the technician is with the slide preparation. Conidia may be in chains or broken apart, with a flat appearance at one end where they were attached (Figure 5.20).

Fusarium spp. are not seen too often. However, it is important to recognize this contaminant because it produces conidia that closely resemble the macroconidia of *Microsporum* spp. *Fusarium* spp. colonies are whitish with a light purple tinge in the center and have a wooly texture. The banana- or boomerang-shaped conidia have a slight bend on the longitudinal axis and three to five transverse septae (Larone 2002).

Penicillium spp. colonies start out small, white, and dense, but within a day or two the center of the colony will turn a characteristic blue/green color. The conidia resemble a paint brush or pitchfork (Figures 5.21 and 5.22).

Mucor and *Rhizopus* spp. are very similar in appearance. The colony color can range from white to gray to brown and the texture is either wooly or cottony. They produce a stalk with a large round capsule containing multiple small spores. It is often described as a lollipop. When making slides, the capsule may break and one may only see a dome-shaped structure at the top of a stalk.

Malassezia spp. and other yeast contaminants may grow on DTM as well. Yeast colonies are typically mucoid or creamy in texture and color can be yellow, orange, pink, or red (Figure 5.23). Some yeast species produce pseudohyphae with oval to round cells that may be budding. *Malassezia* spp. are part of the normal flora of dog and cat skin, so growth on culture does not indicate disease.

Safety Precautions

Dermatophytosis is contagious and zoonotic, therefore special care should be taken when handling and examining fungal cultures. When working with inoculated cultures, always wear exam gloves and a lab coat or other protective attire. Tie back long hair and

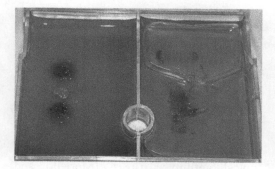

Figure 5.23 Several colonies of yeast, mucoid in texture.

have an area designated for examination of fungal culture plates, preferably away from where patients are examined. Do not interrupt fungal culture examination to perform other tasks. This will minimize contamination of other surfaces and objects. Do not sniff the fungal cultures. Some identification text books describe what the colonies may smell like, but it is not recommended to open the plate and breathe in any spores! Clean the working area with a fungicidal disinfectant, for example a 1:10 bleach solution or accelerated hydrogen peroxide, allowing a minimum contact time of 10 minutes. Do not eat or drink in the immediate area, wash your hands well when done, and discard cultures into the appropriate biohazard containers.

If the fungal cultures need to be shipped to a referral laboratory for identification, be aware of the state's as well as the courier's requirements for the shipment of potentially infectious substances.

Biopsy/Histopathology

Skin biopsies may occasionally be needed to diagnose dermatophytosis when nodular lesions or other unusual presentations occur. Small, single nodules can be completely excised, but if lesions are widespread, multiple 6–8 mm punch biopsy samples should be taken. The veterinarian should include a detailed history on the submission form and should let the pathologist know if dermatophytosis is suspected.

Special histopathological stains such as Gomori methamine silver and periodic acid-Schiff can facilitate the identification of fungal hyphae in tissue samples.

Polymerase Chain Reaction Test

A polymerase chain reaction (PCR) test for the diagnosis of dermatophytosis in dogs and cats has become commercially available in the United States, the Idexx Laboratories Ringworm (Dermatophytosis) RealPCR® test (Westbrook, ME). This detects the presence of DNA from *M. canis*, *Microsporum* spp., and *Trichophyton* spp. in samples of hair, skin scale, and material aspirated from nodular lesions (Idexx 2017). Results from this PCR test are typically available in one to three business days. This rapid turnaround time allows treatment of dermatophytosis to begin sooner than in the past. The author still recommends fungal culture in addition to the PCR testing to identify the species of dermatophyte involved, in case the PCR test identifies *Microsporum* spp. or *Trichophyton* spp. and not *M. canis*. The usefulness of this PCR test to confirm successful resolution of dermatophytosis remains to be evaluated. The PCR test identifies DNA from dermatophytes, but cannot distinguish live from dead dermatophytes, so could potentially be still positive even when treatment is successful. If the PCR test is negative, the clinician can be even more confident that the infection has been cleared.

Treatment

Dermatophytosis can be a self-limiting disease in otherwise healthy dogs and cats, with resolution often occurring within three to four months (Miller et al. 2013a; Moriello and DeBoer 2012). Treatment is still recommended due to the contagious and zoonotic nature of dermatophytosis. Treatment shortens the course of infection, thereby decreasing disease transmission to other pets and people, as well as environmental contamination with infectious arthrospores. Both oral and topical therapy for the patient, plus cleaning of the environment, should be employed. All in-contact pets should be cultured and treated at least topically. Treatment can last several months and should be continued until the patient has at least two consecutive negative fungal cultures (Moriello and DeBoer 2014). Culturing should be done weekly and clients can be taught to collect toothbrush samples from pets at home. The first negative culture may be seen as early as two to three weeks after the start of therapy, so weekly culturing can shorten treatment duration (Moriello and DeBoer 2014). Patients may look clinically normal before they have negative fungal cultures, so clients should be instructed to continue therapy until negative cultures are obtained. If it is possible, affected animals should be confined to areas of the house that can be easily cleaned. Social interaction should be maintained, especially for kittens and puppies, even when they are restricted to certain areas of the house.

Topical Therapy

Clipping removes infected hairs from the patient and decreases contamination of the environment. In long-haired patients clipping also makes topical therapy easier and more effective by ensuring better penetration of the topical agent. The amount of clipping that should be done varies with each patient. Patients with mild or localized disease may only need the hair surrounding the lesions clipped with scissors. Patients with long hair or extensive disease may need whole body clipping. Whole body clipping should be done very carefully with a #10 blade and care should be taken to avoid thermal injury to the skin. Clients should be warned that clinical signs may temporarily worsen after whole body clipping. Clipping should be done in an enclosed room that can be thoroughly cleaned, and a separate set of clippers and blades designated only for dermatophyte patients should be used. Personnel

involved should wear protective clothing that can be discarded or laundered, including caps, gowns, gloves, and shoe covers.

Topical therapy kills infective spores on the haircoat and this decreases environmental contamination. Whole body treatment rather than spot treatment of lesions is recommended (Moriello and DeBoer 2012, 2014).

Lime sulfur and enilconazole (not available in the United States) are the most effective topical antifungal rinses (Moriello and DeBoer 2012, 2014). Miconazole combined with chlorhexidine in a shampoo formulation (Malaseb®, Bayer, Shawnee Mission, KS) has also shown good efficacy against dermatophytes (Moriello and DeBoer 2012). Twice-weekly whole body therapy is recommended (Moriello and DeBoer 2012, 2014). Lime sulfur is very safe and is the best option for very young patients, geriatric animals, or patients that cannot tolerate systemic therapy. Its disadvantages include a bad odor (rotten eggs), yellow staining of light-colored hair, staining of porcelain and other surfaces, and tarnishing jewelry. Communication with owners is essential when dealing with this product, especially if they will be performing the dip at home (see the handout in Box 5.1). Dipping should be done outdoors or in a well-ventilated area. Remove any jewelry and watches before performing the dip and wear gloves and protective clothing. Patients do not need to be bathed before dipping unless they are excessively dirty. If they are bathed first, towel dry before applying the dip. Dilute as directed on label (8 oz of dip in 128 oz (1 gal) of warm water), then sponge dip on the animal until the haircoat is thoroughly saturated. Be sure to treat all areas, including the face and ear pinnae. Remove excess dip solution by gently squeegeeing the animal with both hands so the pet is not dripping wet. Then allow the pet to air dry in a holding cage or carrier (Figure 5.24). If the animal is inclined to groom during the drying period, an Elizabethan collar should be used. Be particularly careful to avoid hypothermia when dipping kittens and puppies.

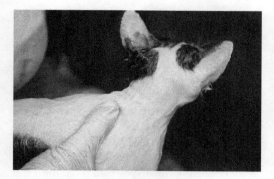

Figure 5.24 Lime sulfur treatment applied to a feline patient. *Source:* Courtesy of Amelia G. White, DVM, MS, DACVD, Auburn University, Auburn, AL.

An alternative method for dipping cats is to use a half-gallon rose sprayer. Keep the nozzle close to the cat's skin when applying the dip so the entire haircoat becomes saturated. Use a sponge or cloth to apply dip to the face and ears. Avoid getting lime sulfur into the eyes. The rose sprayer method is also useful with fractious cats, since this technique can be used through a wire carrier. (Dane County Humane Society 2019).

Enilconazole (Imaverol®, Janssen Pharmaceutica, Mississauga, Ontario, Canada) is another very effective topical antifungal rinse. It is only approved for use on dogs and is not available in the United States. It can be used off-label in cats as long as an Elizabethan collar is used to avoid potential toxicity from the cat ingesting the rinse while grooming (Moriello and DeBoer 2012). Follow label directions for dilution to make a 0.2% solution of enilconazole and apply in the same manner as lime sulfur.

Systemic Antifungals

Systemic antifungal therapy speeds resolution of dermatophytosis for the patient, thereby decreasing the spread of the disease to others. Currently available oral antifungal agents include itraconazole, terbinafine, fluconazole, ketoconazole, and griseofulvin.

Itraconazole (Sporonox®, Janssen) is the recommended therapy due to its effectiveness and low incidence of adverse effects.

The drug's high cost is its primary drawback. Pulse dosing of one week on followed by one week off can be used to decrease drug expense, since itraconazole accumulates in the hair and skin (Moriello and DeBoer, 2012, 2014). Itraconazole comes in a capsule form and oral solution. The oral solution is better absorbed than the capsules and is labeled for use in cats in Europe, and has recently become available in the United States as well (Itrafungol®, Elanco, Greenfield, IN). Itraconazole should be given with food to enhance its absorption. The 100 mg capsules can be opened and the contents divided into smaller doses by mixing with a small amount of butter or food. The human brand-name or generic product can be used, but avoid use of the powdered form of itraconazole available from many compounding pharmacies. The powdered form of the drug is not well absorbed and treatment failures have been reported (Mawby et al. 2014).

Terbinafine is becoming a more popular choice for treatment of dermatophytosis due to the low cost of the generic formulation (Moriello and DeBoer 2012, 2014). The effectiveness of pulse therapy with this drug has not been well documented, so daily dosing is currently recommended. Increases in alanine aminotransferase have been seen, so monitoring of liver enzymes is recommended, particularly for cats (Moriello and DeBoer 2012).

Ketoconazole should not be used in cats (high incidence of hepatotoxicity), and its use in dogs would be recommended only if itraconazole and terbinafine are not an option due to expense or drug intolerance (Moriello and DeBoer 2014).

Fluconazole may be less effective than itraconazole or terbinafine, so this drug would also be a second choice for treating dermatophytosis (Moriello and DeBoer 2014).

Griseofulvin is an old systemic medication for dermatophytosis. It is rarely used due to its potential adverse effects (teratogenicity, vomiting, diarrhea, bone marrow suppression) and the availability of safer and more effective alternatives.

Lufenuron is an inhibitor of chitin synthesis that is marketed as an oral flea control agent. One initial uncontrolled study reported successful treatment of dermatophytosis, but subsequent controlled clinical trials have demonstrated a lack of efficacy (Moriello and DeBoer 2014). Therefore its use is not recommended.

There is also no currently available effective vaccine for the treatment or prevention of dermatophytosis.

Environment

Elimination of dermatophyte spores from the environment is best accomplished with a three step approach (Dane County Humane Society 2019). Removal of hair, dirt, and debris first, followed by cleaning with a detergent and water, and, last, application of a fungicidal disinfectant. Cleaning should be done twice a week. Use of electrostatic dusting cloths (Swiffer®, Procter & Gamble, Cincinnati, OH) and vacuuming are recommended over sweeping to avoid stirring up hair and spores. Vacuum bags should be discarded after each use. Hard surfaces should be washed twice with a detergent solution and then rinsed well. Newer studies show disinfectants labeled as effective against *Trichophyton* spp. can be used to kill spores of *M. canis*. A variety of household disinfectants can be used. Accelerated hydrogen peroxide (Rescue™, Virox Technologies, Ontario, Canada) is gaining in popularity as a fungicide due to its ease of use, lack of strong odor, 5–10 minute contact time, and user safety (Moriello and DeBoer 2014). A 1:100 dilution of household bleach with a 10 minute contact time is also effective, but must be made fresh before each use.

Wash rugs, bed linens, animal bedding, and so on in hot water and dry in a hot dryer. Pet collars, leashes, toys, furniture, and grooming equipment that cannot be laundered should be discarded. Pet carriers should be disinfected and vehicles used for patient transport should be vacuumed thoroughly. Carpeting and fabric-covered furniture can be particularly challenging to clean since most cleaners and disinfectants will discolor the fabric. Thorough vacuuming should be done frequently and patients should not be allowed in these areas if possible. Steam cleaning of carpets does not kill fungal spores unless the water temperature remains above 43.3 °C (170 °F). This temperature cannot be maintained with the machines available for "do-it-yourself" home use (Miller et al. 2013a).

Once the patient is culture negative, the environment should also be cultured to check for any remaining fungal spores. Culturing can be done by wiping surfaces with pieces of Swiffer sweeper cloths and pressing the surface of the cloth onto the fungal culture plate. If there is concern about fungal contamination of heating or cooling ducts, take fungal culture samples from ducts before investing in professional cleaning.

Similar precautions should be taken in the veterinary clinic to minimize fungal contamination. Known or suspect cases of dermatophytosis should come in at the end of the day if possible and should be placed in an examination room immediately to decrease contamination of the waiting room. Smaller pets should be transported in carriers. Protective clothing that can be laundered or discarded should be worn by staff handling the infected patient. Examination rooms should be thoroughly cleaned and disinfected with the same protocol used for disinfection of the home environment. If the room has to be used again that day, it is best to avoid bringing very young, geriatric, sick, or immunosuppressed patients into that room.

Client Education

The amount of information clients must absorb and understand when faced with a diagnosis of dermatophytosis can be overwhelming. The veterinary technician should reinforce and expand on information relayed first by the clinician. Be sure the client understands that dermatophytosis is contagious to other animals as well as people. This will make client compliance with treatment recommendations more likely. Owners should receive detailed instructions for both oral and topical medications prescribed (Box 5.1). If the owner will be dividing itraconazole capsules, they will need to be told or shown how to do this (Box 5.2). Owners may need to be shown how to do toothbrush sampling for fungal cultures. Having a series of handouts with information about the disease, environmental cleaning recommendations, and treatment instructions is extremely useful (Boxes 5.3 and 5.4). The client should understand that their pet will often look clinically normal before the infection is resolved, so recheck appointments are essential and it is a good idea to have the clients schedule the next appointment before they leave the clinic. Complete and thorough client education together with good follow-up will ensure the best compliance and outcome for dermatophytosis patients.

Conclusion

Treatment of dermatophytosis can be difficult, expensive, and lengthy. The veterinary technician can greatly increase the chances of successful management of these cases.

Box 5.1 An example of a topical handout for Lime Sulfur Dip

Lime Sulfur Dip

Directions:

1) Shake Lime Sulfur Dip well.
2) Mix 8 ounces of dip with 1 gallon of warm water. Pour the 8 ounces of dip into the container and then add water to make recommended concentration.
3) Apply solution over your pet's entire body surface; the entire hair coat should be wet to the skin. Then, allow your pet to air dry (outside or in a screened-in area is best). DO NOT RINSE.
4) For cats and small dogs, it may be helpful to fill a bucket, small garbage can or Rubbermaid-type storage bin and dip their bodies in, then sponge over the head/face area.
5) You can also use a half-gallon rose sprayer to apply the dip. Keep the nozzle of the sprayer very close to the skin so the spray flows over your pet like a shower.
6) You can make a portable dip sink by using a laundry sink that drains into a bucket.
7) Lime Sulfur Dip expires in 24 hours once it has been diluted.
8) Repeat treatment twice a week or as directed.

Considerations:

- Dip should be used outside in a well-ventilated area only.
- When using dip, wear gloves and be sure to remove all jewelry.
- Dip will stain/eat through porcelain and stain fabrics.
- Lime Sulfur Dip has a very strong ("rotten egg") odor.
- Dip turns white hair yellowish temporarily.
- Try to keep your pet occupied or place an e-collar (to prevent licking) until your pet is completely dry.
- If your pet becomes red or itchy after a dip, rinse pet several times or bathe with a mild shampoo and call us.
- Ensure entire body/hair coat is thoroughly saturated to the skin.

Should you have any questions or if your pet reacts to the treatment, please call our office. Source: Modified from Dane County Humane Society (2019). Feline Ringworm Treatment Center. https://www.giveshelter.org/our-services/feline-ringworm-treatment-center (accessed May 2019).

Box 5.2 Itraconazole Handout

Itraconazole Administration Instructions

1) Itraconazole (100 mg, regular generic capsules): Give ___ capsule by mouth once daily with food as directed.
2) Make a small tray out of aluminum foil, approximately 1 inch x 2 inches.
3) The capsule is filled with tiny beads. To divide the contents of the capsule, open it and sprinkle onto a small amount of softened butter.
4) Mix thoroughly in order to evenly distribute the beads in the butter.
5) Shape the butter into a rectangle using the foil tray and chill until slightly firm.
6) Divide the butter rectangle into ___ equal pieces and store in the freezer.

Box 5.3 Client Education Handout

Dermatophytosis

What is Dermatophytosis?

- Dermatophytosis, commonly known as ringworm, is a fungal disease of the skin and hair. It is caused by fungi that obtain their nutrients from keratin (skin, hair, and nails).
- Dermatophytosis is contagious to other animals and people.
- If you or a family member has any skin lesions, please contact your physician.

How do animals get Dermatophytosis?

- Dermatophyte infections are transmitted by infected hairs from animals, or by items such as grooming tools or bedding. Dermatophytosis can also be acquired from the environment (for example soil or wild animals).
- The very young, very old, and immunosuppressed individuals are more susceptible to infection.

What are the symptoms of Dermatophytosis?

- Symptoms can vary greatly, but patchy hair loss, reddened skin, scaling, and crusting are often seen.
- Some animals, especially cats, can have very minor lesions that are difficult to find.
- Dermatophytosis is sometimes, but not always itchy.

How is Dermatophytosis diagnosed?

- Dermatophytosis is usually diagnosed by growing the fungus on a culture with samples of hair and skin scale collected from your pet.

How is Dermatophytosis treated?

- Treatment usually includes both oral and topical medication.
- Because dermatophytosis is contagious, all pets in the household will need to be tested and possibly treated.
- Affected animals should be confined to an area of the house that is easily cleaned.
- Treatment may last for several months. Animals may look normal before they are cured, so it is important to continue treatment until at least two consecutive negative fungal cultures have been obtained.
- Fungal spores can survive for a long time in the environment, so cleaning and disinfecting the home environment is an important part of treatment.

Box 5.4 Environmental Cleaning Handout

General Environmental Cleaning for Dermatophytosis

- Fungal spores are primarily hair-borne, so they go where hair and dust go (via floating, drifting, being carried on clothing, etc.). Cat hair gets everywhere!
- If possible, confine pets to easily cleaned rooms. Close closets and drawers and remove knick-knacks.
- Thoroughly dust surfaces with Swiffer-type dusters and vacuum or use Swiffer-type sweepers on floors as often as possible, but at least twice a week.
- Minimize how much you stir up spores through sweeping, flailing bedding about, etc.
- Use electrostatic cleaners such as Swiffers or damp mopping in preference over sweeping whenever possible.
- Wash hard surfaces with detergent and water as often as possible, but at least twice a week.
- Launder (hot water/dryer) rugs, animal bedding, and other pet-contact bed linens.
- Launder, disinfect, or discard pet toys and grooming aids and furniture.
- If possible, disinfect hard surfaces with a product labeled as effective against *Trichophyton* spp. e.g. Rescue™ (accelerated hydrogen peroxide); allow 10 minutes of wetting time.
- Vacuum and disinfect (if possible) any vehicles and transport cages used for animals.

- After animals are clear, obtain culture specimens to check for environmental contamination by wiping small squares of Swiffer cloths over exposed areas and use the surfaces of the cloths to inoculate fungal culture plates.
- Take fungal cultures of ductwork using Swiffer duster cloths before you invest in duct cleaning. You only need to clean if the culture is positive.
- The most effective way to keep the environment clean and to decontaminate the environment is to use the triple cleaning technique:
  a) Mechanical removal of dirt, hair, etc.
  b) Wash the area with detergent and water.
  c) Disinfect with a product labeled as effective against *Trichophyton* spp. e.g. accelerated hydrogen peroxide (Rescue™).

The most important steps are (a) and (b): good old-fashioned house cleaning! Think of spores like dust.

Source: Moriello, K.A. and DeBoer, D.J. (2014). Treatment of dermatophytosis. In Bonagura, J.D. and Twedt, D.C. (eds.), *Kirk's Current Veterinary Therapy XV*, pp. 449–451. Philadelphia, PA: Elsevier Saunders, Box 105-1: Recommended environmental control measures in the treatment of dermatophytosis; cleaning recommendations in Dane County Humane Society (2019). Feline Ringworm Treatment Center. https://www.giveshelter.org/our-services/feline-ringworm-treatment-center (accessed May 2019).

Obtaining an accurate history, recognizing clinical signs, collecting appropriate samples, and correctly identifying dermatophyte species from cultures are all important for the diagnosis of dermatophytosis. Perhaps most important of all is complete and detailed client education. Owners who understand how dermatophytosis is spread will be more likely to adhere to treatment recommendations, both for the pet and for the environment. Taking the time to ensure clients understand all the details of their treatment plan as well as the importance of treating until the patient is culture negative is extremely important. Close follow-up with frequent communication by the veterinary technician can help clients complete therapy and successfully eliminate dermatophytosis.

References

Cornegliani, L., Persico, P., and Colombo, S. (2009). Canine nodular dermatophytosis (kerion): 23 cases. *Veterinary Dermatology* 20: 185–190.

Idexx (2017). Diagnosis and management of dermatophytosis with the Ringworm (Dermatophyte) RealPCRTM Panel. https://www.idexx.com/files/ringworm-pcr-panel.pdf (accessed May 2019).

Larone, D.H. (2002). *Medically Important Fungi: A Guide to Identification*, 4e. Washington, DC: ASM Press.

Logan, M.R., Raskin, R.E., and Thompson, S. (2006). "Carry-on" dermal baggage: a nodule from a dog. *Veterinary Clinical Pathology* 35 (3): 329–331.

Mawby, D.I., Whittemore, J.C., Genger, S., and Papich, M.G. (2014). Bioequivalence of orally administered generic, compounded, and innovato-formulated itraconazole in healthy dogs. *Journal of Veterinary Internal Medicine* 28 (1): 72–77.

Miller, W.H., Griffin, C.E., and Campbell, K.L. (2013a). Fungal and algal skin diseases. In: *Muller & Kirk's Small Animal Dermatology*, 7e (eds. W. Miller, C. Griffin and K. Campbell), 223–283. St. Louis: Elsevier Mosby.

Miller, W.H., Griffin, C.E., and Campbell, K.L. (2013b). Diagnostic methods. In: *Muller & Kirk's Small Animal Dermatology*, 7e (eds. W. Miller, C. Griffin and K. Campbell), 57–107. St. Louis: Elsevier Mosby.

Moriello, K.A. (2016). Dermatophytosis: diagnosis and effective treatment. "This much I know to be true." *Proceedings of the 8th World Congress of Veterinary Dermatology*, June. Bordeaux, France. pp. 238–245.

Moriello, K.A. and DeBoer, D.J. (2012). Dermatophytosis. In: *Infectious Diseases of the Dog and Cat*, 4e (ed. C.E. Greene), 558–602. St. Louis: Elsevier Saunders.

Moriello, K.A. and DeBoer, D.J. (2014). Treatment of Dermatophytosis. In: *Kirk's Current Veterinary Therapy XV* (eds. J.D. Bonagura and D.C. Twedt), 449–451. St. Louis: Elsevier Saunders.

Peters, J.D., Scott, D.W., Erb, H.N. et al. (2007). Comparative analysis of canine dermatophytosis and superficial pemphigus for the prevalence of dermatophyes and acantholytic keratinocytes: a histopathological and clinicial retrospective study. *Veterinary Dermatology* 18: 234–240.

Scott, D.W. and Miller, W.H. Jr. (eds.) (2003). Fungal skin diseases. In: *Equine Dermatology*, 261–320. St. Louis: W.B. Saunders.

Verbrugge, M., Kettings, R., and Moriello, K. (2008). Effects of light and temperature variations on time to growth of dermatophytes using commercial fungal culture media [abstract]. *Veterinary Dermatology* 19: 110.

Recommended Reading

Dane County Humane Society (2019). Feline Ringworm Treatment Center. https://www.giveshelter.org/our-services/feline-ringworm-treatment-center (accessed May 2019).

Moriello, K.A. (2014). Feline dermatophytosis: aspects pertinent to disease management in single and multiple cat situations. *Journal of Feline Medicine and Surgery* 16: 419–431.

Recommended Fungal Identification References

Larone, D.H. (2002). *Medically Important Fungi; A Guide to Identification*, 4e. Washington, DC: ASM Press.

St-Germain, G. and Summerbell, R. (1996). *Identifying Filamentous Fungi: A Clinical Laboratory Handbook*. Belmont, CA: Star Publishing Company.

University of Adelaide (2019). Mycology Online. http://www.mycology.adelaide.edu.au (accessed May 2019).

Section III

Allergic Skin Diseases

6

Flea Allergy Dermatitis
Missy Streicher

Introduction

Flea allergy dermatitis (FAD) is one of the most common allergic skin diseases seen in dogs and cats (Kunkle and Halliwell 2003; Miller et al. 2013). FAD is the result of a hypersensitivity reaction to flea saliva injected into the host when the flea bites. Both immediate (type I) and delayed (type IV) hypersensitivity reactions have been demonstrated in the dog (Kunkle and Halliwell 2003; Miller et al. 2013). With repeated exposure to flea bites, many pets will develop FAD (Kunkle and Halliwell 2003). Non-flea allergic pets can carry a high flea burden without showing significant signs of discomfort, while the exquisitely flea-allergic pet may be intolerant of even a few flea bites.

In addition to causing significant discomfort, fleas can serve as vectors for zoonotic diseases such as typhus, plague, and bartonellosis. Fleas are also the intermediate host for the tapeworm *Dipylidium caninum*. Pets may ingest tapeworm-infected fleas during self-grooming. Tapeworm segments (proglottids) may be seen on the pet's stool, around the pet's anal area or perineum, or on the pet's bedding. Proglottids are often described by owners as looking like grains of rice when they have dried. In areas of the world where fleas are common, the presence of tapeworms is most often indicative of past flea exposure. Severe flea infestations can result in anemia, especially in smaller pets.

The cat flea, *Ctenocephalides felis felis*, is the flea most commonly found on dogs and cats in most areas of the world (Figures 6.1 and 6.2). A thorough knowledge of the biology and life cycle of this flea is essential for developing effective flea control programs. Fleas thrive at temperatures between 20 and 30 °C (68–86 °F) and relative humidity around 70%. An adult cat flea spends its entire life on its host. Female fleas begin laying eggs as soon as 24 hours after they begin feeding, and they are prolific egg producers, laying up to 40–50 eggs daily. Flea eggs and feces fall off the host into the environment. The eggs may be visible as tiny white dots on dark surfaces (Figure 6.3). In 2–10 days the eggs hatch into larvae and proceed through three larval stages (Figure 6.4). The larvae feed on adult flea feces, flea eggs, and other larvae. Flea larvae prefer dark, warm, moist environments such as the base of carpets (Figure 6.5) and shady areas under decks, trees, and shrubs, especially when protected by leaf litter or mulch. When the larvae are ready to pupate in one to three weeks, they spin a cocoon (Figure 6.6). Once inside the cocoon, the pupa transforms into the pre-emergent adult flea that is capable of hatching in as little as five days, or can remain dormant for as long as six months. The pre-emergent adult flea inside its cocoon is protected from the effects of insecticides. The adult flea is stimulated to emerge from the cocoon by heat and

Small Animal Dermatology for Technicians and Nurses, First Edition. Edited by Kim Horne, Marcia Schwassmann and Dawn Logas.

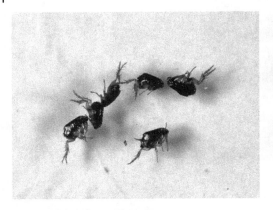

Figure 6.1 Adult fleas (*Ctenocephalides felis*). *Source:* Courtesy of Dr. Byron Blagburn, MS, PhD.

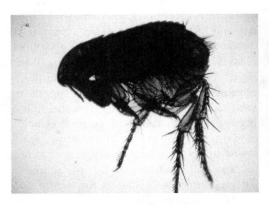

Figure 6.2 Magnified (4×) adult flea (*Ctenocephalides felis*).

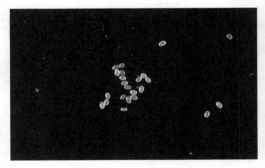

Figure 6.3 Flea eggs. *Source:* Courtesy of Dr. Byron Blagburn, MS, PhD.

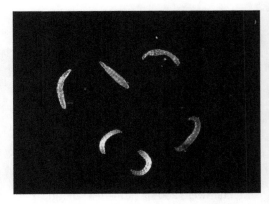

Figure 6.4 Flea larva. *Source:* Courtesy of Dr. Byron Blagburn, MS, PhD.

mechanical pressure that indicate the presence of a suitable host. Under ideal conditions, the flea life cycle can be completed in as little as 14 days (Kunkle and Halliwell 2003; Rust and Dryden 1997). The cat flea is not host specific and uses cats, dogs, ferrets, rabbits, coyotes, foxes, opossums, and raccoons as hosts, so wildlife can be important sources of flea infestations (Kunkle and Halliwell 2003; Rust and Dryden 1997). Fleas multiply rapidly and flea eggs and larvae make up the bulk of the flea population, with adults representing only a small fraction.

Modern flea control products have greatly decreased the time and effort required for successful treatment of flea-allergic pets.

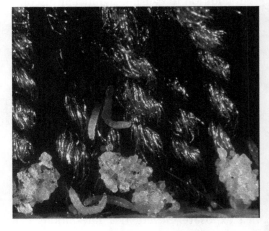

Figure 6.5 Flea stages (egg, larvae, and pupae) in carpet. *Source:* Courtesy of Dr. Byron Blagburn, MS, PhD.

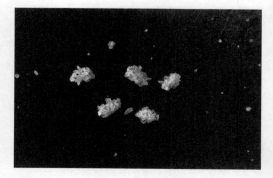

Figure 6.6 Flea pupae. *Source:* Courtesy of Dr. Byron Blagburn, MS, PhD.

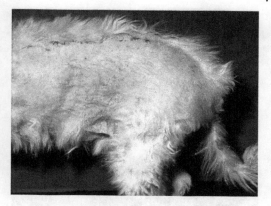

Figure 6.7 Dog with flea allergy dermatitis exhibiting extensive alopecia and folliculitis (secondary pyoderma). *Source:* Courtesy of Dr. Robert Kennis.

However, client education remains critical to the success of flea control programs and the veterinary technician is the ideal person to convey this information. Treatment failures are almost always due to inadequate or incomplete flea control programs rather than resistance to flea adulticides. Clients who have an understanding of the flea life cycle, how flea control products work, and how long it takes to eliminate an infestation will have the best chance for success.

Clinical Features

In dogs, flea allergy presents as a pruritic, papular, erythematous dermatitis typically affecting the caudal half of the body, more specifically the lumbosacral area, caudomedial thighs, dorsal tail head, flanks, and ventral abdomen (Figures 6.7 and 6.8). Self-trauma results in focal or more generalized alopecia and chronic cases can develop hyperpigmentation, lichenification, and fibropruritic nodules (Figure 6.9). Pyotraumatic dermatitis, bacterial folliculitis, and malassezia dermatitis often occur secondary to FAD (Kunkle and Halliwell 2003; Miller et al. 2013).

FAD in cats has a variety of clinical presentations, including non-inflammatory alopecia, erythema, papules, crusted papules (miliary dermatitis), and the eosinophilic granuloma complex (Figures 6.10 and 6.11). Lesions may be found almost anywhere on

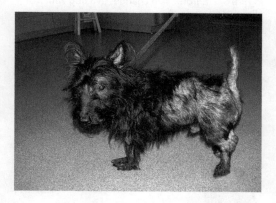

Figure 6.8 Dog with caudal patchy alopecia secondary to flea allergy dermatitis.

the body, but are most commonly present on the head, ventral abdomen and inguinal area, caudal dorsum, and tail (Favrot 2014; Logas 2014; Miller et al. 2013). Most cats with FAD are pruritic and owners will note scratching, chewing, and increased grooming behavior; however, some cats will only over-groom when they are not observed. Owners may present these cats for hair loss and will insist the patient is not pruritic. A trichogram is the best way to determine if the alopecia is self-induced. Hairs that have been groomed off will have blunted, broken-off ends instead of the normal shaft that tapers to a point (Figures 6.12 and 6.13). While this is not

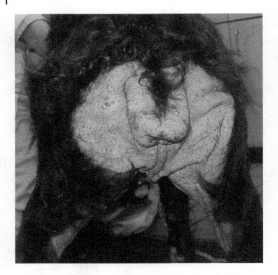

Figure 6.9 Chronic skin changes in a dog with flea allergy dermatitis.

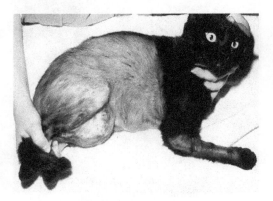

Figure 6.10 Cat with flea allergy dermatitis. *Source:* Courtesy of Dr. Robert Kennis.

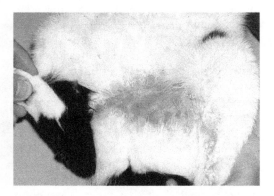

Figure 6.11 Cat with eosinophilic plaque secondary to flea allergy dermatitis. *Source:* Courtesy of Dr. Robert Kennis.

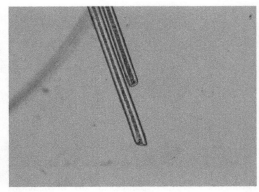

Figure 6.12 Trichogram illustrating broken hairs from traumatically induced alopecia in a flea-allergic cat; note the blunted ends of the hairs.

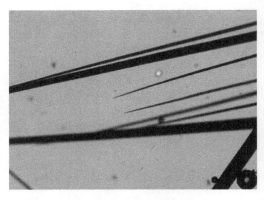

Figure 6.13 Trichogram illustrating the tapered ends of hairs in a cat with a normal hair coat.

diagnostic for flea allergy, it may indicate traumatically induced alopecia secondary to pruritus from FAD.

No breed or sex predilections have been observed for FAD. Flea bite hypersensitivity can occur at any age, but in flea-endemic areas clinical signs usually develop by five years of age (Miller et al. 2013). The patient's age at onset of signs is probably more dependent on degree of prior flea exposure. Clinical signs may be seasonal in colder climates, but are often year round in temperate and tropical zones, where temperature and humidity support flea survival year round.

FAD can occur together with atopic dermatitis and food hypersensitivities; therefore, flea exposure can cause clinical signs that may be misinterpreted as a flare-up of a concurrent allergy. Also, there is evidence that atopic dermatitis predisposes to the development of FAD (Sousa and Halliwell 2001). This further emphasizes the need for maintaining year-round flea control for patients with atopic dermatitis.

It is not unusual for owners to fail to see fleas on their flea allergic pets. Flea allergic individuals can be extremely efficient at grooming off fleas, therefore the absence of fleas on a patient does not rule out a diagnosis of FAD (Kunkle and Halliwell 2003; Miller et al. 2013). Clients may be reluctant to acknowledge that their pet has fleas. They may feel the presence of fleas implies they are not caring for their pets properly or that they are living in unsanitary conditions. The veterinary technician can help correct these misconceptions by teaching clients about flea biology and the flea life cycle. The veterinary technician can also help the client understand that instituting strict flea control is necessary to rule out FAD as a differential diagnosis.

Diagnostic Tests

A history of flea exposure in a patient with compatible clinical signs strongly supports a diagnosis of FAD, and this diagnosis is confirmed by a positive response to stringent flea control (Kunkle and Halliwell 2003; Miller et al. 2013). The dermatological history (see Chapter 1) can guide the clinician in determining the likelihood of FAD as a diagnosis. The history should include information on clinical signs such as presence of pruritus, location and degree of pruritus, lesion description, lesion location, age of pet at onset of signs, duration of signs, and seasonality of signs. Owners should be asked if they have seen fleas on the patient as well as on any other pets in the household. Information about the patient's environment is also important. Owners should be asked if pets are housed indoors or outdoors and if they are allowed to roam freely outdoors. The presence of other pets in the household, stray dogs and cats, and wildlife should be documented. The nature of the indoor environment, for instance carpeting versus hard flooring, and the outdoor conditions, for example shady yard versus open and sunny yard, should be noted, as they can have an impact on flea control recommendations. Details about current flea control measures such as which products are used, how often they are used, and whether all pets in the household are treated are also important.

Physical examination may reveal the presence of fleas or flea feces (commonly called "flea dirt") on the pet. Using a flea comb may increase the chances of finding adult fleas and flea feces. Adult fleas are small, brown, laterally compressed, wingless ectoparasites that can jump great distances. Flea feces are usually small, dry particles, dark brown to black in color (Figure 6.14). Placing the "flea dirt" on a moistened paper towel or gauze pad will turn the towel red to a reddish brown, revealing the digested blood that makes up flea fecal material (Figure 6.15). The presence of "flea dirt" on the pet demonstrates that a flea has been on the pet long enough to take a blood meal and to defecate, which might help disprove the often-stated client assertion that the pet

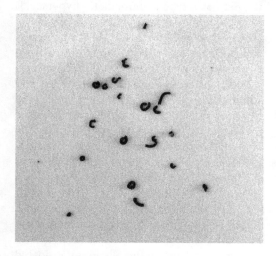

Figure 6.14 Dry flea feces. *Source:* Courtesy of Dr. Byron Blagburn, MS, PhD.

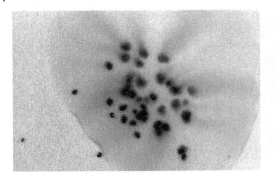

Figure 6.15 Flea feces moistened on a towel. Note the red appearance due to the blood present in the flea feces. *Source:* Courtesy of Dr. Byron Blagburn, MS, PhD.

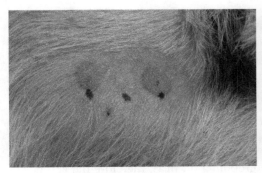

Figure 6.16 Intradermal allergy test demonstrating a positive reaction to flea antigen in a dog. From left to right, the allergens above the marker dot are histamine (positive control), saline (negative control), and flea antigen.

must have just now acquired those fleas at the veterinary establishment. Keep in mind that the absence of fleas or flea feces does not rule out a diagnosis of FAD. Failure to respond to stringent flea control is the only way to definitively rule out a flea allergy.

Intradermal testing with flea antigen can be a useful way to demonstrate flea hypersensitivity to an owner. A positive control (histamine), a negative control (saline), and flea antigen are injected intradermally on a small area of the lateral thorax that has been clipped free of hair. This procedure can usually be performed without sedation. The development of an erythematous wheal at the site of the flea antigen injection indicates the pet has a type I (immediate) hypersensitivity reaction to flea bites (Figure 6.16). However, a negative result does not necessarily rule out flea allergy. Type I (immediate) hypersensitivity reactions can be suppressed by corticosteroids and antihistamines, and some patients exhibit only a delayed-type hypersensitivity reaction. It is therefore important to have owners watch the skin test area for 24–48 hours and report the development of erythema, swelling, and crusting at the injection site (Kunkle and Halliwell 2003; Miller et al. 2013).

Measurement of serum immunoglobulin E (IgE) levels to flea antigens is available as an individual test or as part of a larger panel. Serological testing for flea allergy is considered less reliable than intradermal testing, since it can only detect IgE-dependent reactions (type I hypersensitivity). Serology will not detect flea allergic individuals who have only a delayed-type hypersensitivity. The method of collection (blood draw), expense, and time to get the results of the test also limit the popularity of serum testing for flea allergy. Skin biopsies are not particularly useful for the diagnosis of FAD, as histopathology of suspected lesions tends to be non-specific (Kunkle and Halliwell 2003; Miller et al. 2013).

Treatment

The treatment of FAD involves alleviating pruritus, treating any secondary infections, and avoiding flea bites as much as possible. Patients may need short courses of glucocorticoids or oclacitinib for temporary relief of pruritus while flea control measures are instituted. Oral antibiotics and antifungals may be needed for patients with severe infections. Failure to recognize and treat secondary infection can result in incomplete resolution of signs despite rigorous flea control. Topical therapy with antimicrobial and antipruritic agents can also be beneficial.

The goals of a flea control program are to kill adult fleas on the pet, kill immature flea stages in the environment, and prevent reinfestations. Many highly effective flea adulticides, both topical and oral, are available today. It is expected that by the time of publication of this book, many new flea and tick control products will be available. The reader should be familiar with all the products their veterinary establishment recommends. Currently available topically applied adulticides include pyrethrins, pyrethroids (synthetic pyrethrins), imidacloprid, fipronil, selamectin, dinotefuran, spinetoram, indoxacarb, and fluralaner. Orally administered adulticides include nitenpyram, spinosad, afoxalaner, fluralaner, and sarolaner. Most topical products are available as spot-on formulations, and pyrethrins, pyrethroids, and fipronil are also available as sprays. The spot-on formulations contain vehicles that enable the active ingredient to spread out from the application site to cover the entire animal. Some of these topical agents have activity against other ectoparasites in addition to fleas.

Pyrethrins and pyrethroids (synthetic pyrethrins) are the oldest compounds in this group. Pyrethrin is a natural insecticide produced from the chrysanthemum flower. It has very low toxicity, but its rapid inactivation by ultraviolet light necessitates frequent application. Most pyrethroids are more photostable. Examples of pyrethroids include permethrin, resmethrin, allethrin, deltamethrin, tetramethrin, flumethrin, cyphenothrin, and fenvalerate (Miller et al. 2013; Environmental Protection Agency 2019). These compounds have good activity against adult fleas, ticks, lice, flies, mosquitoes, ear mites (*Otodectes cynotis*), *Cheyletiella* spp., and cat fur mites (*Lynxacarus radovsky*); (Kennis 2004; Miller et al. 2013). Pyrethrins and pyrethroids also have some repellent activity against fleas, mosquitoes, and *Culicoides* spp. (Kunkle and Halliwell 2003). Pyrethroids are frequently found in combination with another flea adulticide as a spot-on product. Examples of these combination products include dinotefuran with permethrin, imidacloprid with permethrin, and fipronil with cyphenothrin. Low concentrations (0.05–0.2%) of pyrethrins are relatively safe in cats, but the higher concentrations of pyrethroids used on dogs can be extremely toxic to cats (Kunkle and Halliwell 2003; Miller et al. 2013), therefore great care should be taken to avoid accidental application of products labeled for use on dogs to cats. Flumethrin is the only pyrethroid safe for use in cats. It is available in combination with imidacloprid in a long-acting flea and tick collar that is labeled for use in dogs and cats.

Imidacloprid was one of the first of the new generation of flea adulticides to be released. It is a chloronicotinyl nitroguanidine (neonicotinoid) insecticide with good activity against adult fleas and some flea larvicidal activity (Jacobs et al. 2001). It has also been shown to have activity against lice in dogs (Mencke 2000). Imidacloprid is available in combination with moxidectin as a spot-on formulation. Moxidectin is an avermectin that prevents heartworm disease and has activity against intestinal parasites (hookworms, roundworms, whipworms), ear mites, scabies mites, demodex mites, and lice (Burrows 2009). The label-approved uses of these combination products vary by country, so careful review of all product information is recommended before use. Imidacloprid is also available in combination with the insect growth regulator pyriproxyfen, and for dogs there is a spot-on containing imidacloprid and permethrin, as well as a spot-on containing imidacloprid, permethrin, and pyriproxyfen. The permethrin provides repellant activity against ticks, mosquitoes, and biting flies (Kennis 2004). Imidacloprid in combination with flumethrin (pyrethroid) has recently become available in a collar for use on dogs and cats. The active ingredients are embedded in the polymer matrix of the collar. This provides a continuous slow release of the compounds that protects against fleas and ticks for up to eight months. The collar is labeled for use in both dogs and cats due to flumethrin's unique position as the only pyrethroid currently used for flea and tick control that is safe for cats.

Fipronil is a phenylpyrazole insecticide that was released as a spot-on formulation shortly after imidacloprid. Fipronil has activity against adult fleas and ticks, as well as scabies mites (*Sarcoptes scabiei*) and chewing lice, *Trichodectes canis* in dogs, and *Felicola subrostratus* in cats. It is available as a spray, a spot-on product, and in combination with the insect growth regulator methoprene as a spot-on product. Fipronil with cyphenothrin and fipronil with amitraz are available as spot-on formulations for dogs. Cyphenothrin, a pyrethroid, and amitraz, a formamidine pesticide, provide increased efficacy against ticks.

Dinotefuran is a newer neonicotinoid insecticide approved for flea control. It has good activity against adult fleas and is available as a spot-on formulation in combination with the insect growth regulator pyriproxyfen. Dinotefuran is also available in combination with pyriproxyfen and permethrin as a spot-on formulation for dogs only. The permethrin provides activity against ticks, mosquitoes, lice, sand flies, and biting flies.

Spinetoram is a member of the spinosyn class of insecticides available as a topical spot-on for cats. It has activity against adult fleas. Indoxacarb is a novel oxadiazone insecticide with activity against adult fleas and flea larvae. This compound has very low mammalian toxicity since it is activated by enzymes in the flea midgut (Merck Animal Health 2012). Indoxacarb is available as a spot-on formulation for dogs and cats, and in combination with permethrin as a spot-on for dogs only.

Selamectin is a topically applied spot-on that also acts systemically. It is absorbed into the bloodstream and then redistributes to the skin. This avermectin has activity against adult fleas, as well as being larvicidal and ovicidal (McTier et al. 2000). Selamectin is also a heartworm preventative and controls ear mites (*O. cynotis*). In dogs it is labeled for control of sarcoptic mange and tick infestations with *Dermacentor variabilis*. In cats it is labeled for control of the roundworm *Toxacara cati* and the hookworm *Ancylostoma tubaeforme*. Since selamectin treats sarcoptic mange in dogs, one might expect it also to control notoedric mange in cats.

Nitenpyram is an orally administered neonicotinoid insecticide. It is approved for use in dogs and cats and provides effective flea adulticide activity that lasts 48 hours (Rust et al. 2003). Because of its rapid onset of action, it is often used as an adjunct to other flea control products when a pet experiences a flea infestation or goes to locations where it may be exposed to fleas. Nitenpyram has been shown to be safe when used together with imidacloprid, fipronil, pyrethrins, and lufenuron (Novartis Animal Health NADA 141–175 Capstar® Nitenpyram).

Spinosad is an orally administered spinosyn insecticide with activity against adult fleas. It is approved for use in dogs and cats. It is given once a month and should be administered with a meal to ensure good absorption of the drug. Spinosad is available in combination with milbemycin for heartworm, flea, and intestinal parasite (*Ancylostoma caninum, Toxocara canis, Toxascaris leonina, Trichuris vulpis*) control in dogs. Spinosad should not be used concurrently in dogs receiving daily high-dose ivermectin for the treatment of generalized demodicosis, due to reports of reactions consistent with ivermectin toxicosis (Elanco 2018; Koch et al. 2012).

Afoxalaner (NexGard®), fluralaner (Bravecto®), and sarolaner (Simparica®) are recently released isoxazoline insecticides with activity against adult fleas and ticks. Afoxalaner and sarolaner are approved for once-a-month use in dogs. Fluralaner is approved for administration once every three months and is available as an oral chewable for dogs, as well as a topical formulation for dogs and cats.

The insect growth regulators methoprene and pyriproxyfen are flea juvenile hormone analogs that stop the development of flea larvae. They are extremely safe for mammals and are available for on-pet application and environmental use. Methoprene is inactivated by sunlight, limiting its usefulness outdoors. Indoors it remains effective for several months. Pyriproxyfen is resistant to ultraviolet radiation, so it can be used indoors and outdoors; however, outdoor use is not recommended due to concern about its persistence in the outdoor environment and possible undesirable effects on beneficial insects (Kunkle and Halliwell 2003; Miller et al. 2013).

The insect development inhibitor lufenuron is a benzoylphenyl urea derivative that inhibits chitin synthesis. Chitin forms the exoskeleton of fleas and without it, flea eggs do not hatch, flea larvae do not develop, and flea pupae are unable to emerge from their cocoons. Lufenuron has no activity against adult fleas. It is available as a once-a-month tablet for dogs and cats, a once-a-month liquid for cats, and a six-month injectable formulation for cats. The tablets and liquid should be given with a meal to ensure adequate absorption of the drug. Lufenuron is available in combination with milbemycin, and with milbemycin and praziquantel for once-a-month administration for heartworm prevention, intestinal parasite control, and control of flea populations in dogs.

Control of flea egg and larval populations in the environment is an important and often neglected part of a complete flea control program. This can be accomplished by mechanical means, on-pet products, and premise treatments. Regular vacuuming of carpets can remove large numbers of eggs and larvae (Kunkle and Halliwell 2003; Rust and Dryden 1997). Remember to properly dispose of the vacuumed contents immediately after each use, or the flea larvae and eggs will develop and contribute to a continuing infestation. Placing the vacuum bag into the freezer will kill the eggs and larvae. Raking up leaf litter and mulch and increasing sun exposure in outdoor environments can also be helpful (Kunkle and Halliwell 2003). Blocking off access to shaded, protected areas underneath decks or porches is recommended. Client handouts explaining the flea life cycle and the flea control process in detail are helpful educational tools (Boxes 6.1 and 6.2).

Once a flea infestation has been eliminated, flea control measures must be continued to prevent future problems. Most pets are at risk for new flea exposure, so year-round or at least seasonal flea control measures are necessary.

Client Education

The veterinary technician plays a central role in educating pet owners about flea control and the treatment of FAD. Setting realistic expectations for product performance is an important part of the treatment of this disease. Providing detailed instructions on how to properly use flea control products will help improve compliance. Since treatment failures are often related to client factors, the veterinary technician must explain the goals of treatment: killing the adult fleas and treating the patient for any secondary infections, eliminating the immature flea stages that exist in the environment, and selecting preventative measures for the future.

Flea control programs must be tailored to each individual pet and client. Oral products may be more effective for pets that swim or are bathed frequently, and clients with small children may prefer oral products to minimize human contact with insecticides. The patient's need for other insect bite, such as mosquito, avoidance and the patient's potential for exposure to other ectoparasites such as ticks and mites, will also influence the veterinarian's choice of flea control products.

Good client communication is essential to successful flea control. The entire veterinary team must have a thorough understanding of flea biology as well as the flea control products they recommend. Simply handing a client a flea adulticide without additional information or instructions is a recipe for failure. Once the veterinarian has decided which products to recommend for the patient, the veterinary technician can then go over details of the customized flea control program with the client (Box 6.3).

A brief review of the flea life cycle and flea biology is a good starting point. Be sure the client understands that if they are seeing adult fleas on the pet, these fleas came from

---

Box 6.1 Example of a Client Handout Explaining the Flea Life Cycle and Flea Control

Fleas and Flea Control for your Pet

Flea allergy dermatitis is a common skin disease of dogs and cats. In addition to causing serious discomfort, fleas can transmit diseases to both people and pets. Flea control is key to the successful treatment of flea-allergic patients and knowing a few facts about the flea life cycle is a tremendous aid in the battle against fleas.

Newly hatched adult fleas jump onto a host (your dog or cat) and stay there. Adult fleas live for approximately 4 months and females can lay up to 40–50 eggs daily.

The eggs are not sticky and fall off the host animal into the environment. The highest concentration of eggs will be found in areas where your pet spends the most time. The eggs hatch in 2–10 days and are now in the larval stage.

Flea larvae prefer dark, warm, moist areas such as the base of carpets, and shady, protected areas outdoors, e.g., under decks, sheds, mulch or leaf litter. In another 1–3 weeks when they are ready to pupate, the larvae spin a cocoon. In a process similar to the caterpillar's transformation into a butterfly, the larva turns into the adult flea.

The adult flea can hatch in as little as 5 days or can remain dormant for up to 6 months and the cocoon protects the flea inside it from the effects of pesticides. This ability of the pre-emergent adult flea to remain dormant inside its protective cocoon is why complete flea control can take 3–4 months to achieve. Flea populations grow rapidly and under ideal conditions, the flea life cycle can be completed in as little as 2 weeks.

In any given population of fleas, immature stages (eggs and larvae) make up about 95% of the population and adult fleas make up only about 5% of the population. This means that for every adult flea you see on your pet, there are MANY more eggs and larvae in your environment. Wildlife (particularly opossums, raccoons, foxes, coyotes) carry fleas and untreated neighborhood animals or strays may be bringing fleas and their eggs into your yard.

The goals of a flea control program are to kill adult fleas on your pet(s), kill immature flea stages in the environment, and prevent re-infestations. All pets in the household must be treated, not just the flea-allergic individual. Professional exterminators or the do-it-yourself approach may be used for environmental treatment. All areas of the indoor environment your pet has access to must be treated, including under beds, under other furniture, and inside closets. Regular vacuuming of carpets can remove large numbers of eggs and larvae. Replace vacuum bags after each use and dispose of used vacuum bags in a sealed container.

Outdoor environmental control measures should concentrate on areas suitable for flea larval development that your pet frequents. Sunny areas of the yard without protective leaf litter or mulch are not favorable for flea larval development. Shady areas under decks or porches should be blocked off or the area should be treated. Shady areas under trees and bushes should also be treated. Depending on geographical location and seasonality, these steps may not always be needed as fleas do not survive in freezing temperatures.

Remember that complete flea control takes several months. Stick with your program and please call us if you have any questions or concerns. Together we can eliminate fleas and make your pet comfortable again.

---

eggs that were deposited in the environment several weeks ago. Pets typically acquire newly hatched fleas, since adult fleas seldom jump from one host to another (Kunkle and Halliwell 2003). The client must also understand that for every adult flea they see, there are many more eggs and larvae in the environment. Be sure to tell clients it will take

---

Box 6.2 Example of a Client Handout Explaining "Do-it-Yourself" Premise Flea Control

"Do-it-Yourself" Premise Flea Control

Inside the Home
Observe where your pet spends most of his/ her time, and this is where the largest amount of flea eggs will be. Cats in particular have favorite out-of-the-way areas to hide (under the bed, in a closet, etc.) that will need to be treated with a pesticide, otherwise a re-infestation will soon occur. Thorough vacuuming of carpeted areas is recommended before treating. Vacuuming removes a good percentage of flea eggs and larvae from the carpet, stimulates pre-emergent adults to hatch which makes them susceptible to the insecticide, and lifts the carpet strands up so that the spray can penetrate deeper into the carpet. Move furniture and vacuum underneath. Immediately after vacuuming is completed, discard the vacuum cleaner contents in a sealed container or freeze it. Otherwise the eggs and larvae will continue to develop into adult fleas which are able to crawl out of the bag and re-infest the home.

Severe infestations may require use of a product that contains a flea adulticide as well as an insect growth regulator. Insect growth regulators stop the development of flea eggs and larvae. The pyrethrins and synthetic pyrethrins, e.g., permethrin, resmethrin, allethrin, cyfluthrin, fenvalerate, are commonly used to kill adult fleas. Methoprene and pyroproxifen are the commonly used insect growth regulators. They are stable in the indoor environment for several months. Fleas that are already in the pupal stage when the product is applied will not be affected by the chemical and will eventually hatch. This can cause a re-infestation 1–2 weeks after the initial treatment is applied. A second application of the chosen product may be necessary.

Foggers are good for covering large areas, but they do not provide good treatment of areas underneath furniture. A hand-held sprayer can be used in conjunction with foggers or by itself. A hand-held sprayer may be more effective for flea control as it can be directed to areas that need targeting the most. Be sure to spray underneath furniture. Flea larvae prefer dark, moist areas so be sure to spray in corners, under beds, and in closets. When cats are in the household, the entire house needs to be treated as cats are able to access virtually the entire home. Always thoroughly read the manufacturer's recommendations for proper application techniques, reapplication protocols, and precautions or contraindications for use, as other species such as birds or fish may be sensitive to the product.

Wash pet bedding in hot water weekly. If your pet spends time on furniture that cannot be washed, or if your pet travels frequently in vehicles, vacuum areas thoroughly and discard vacuum bags as described earlier. Use caution when spraying pesticides in vehicles as passengers may not tolerate the chemicals.

Yard Treatment
Most flea eggs and larvae do not survive in areas with direct sun exposure. Outdoor flea control efforts should concentrate on shady, protected areas. Keep the lawn mowed, rake leaves, and discard the yard debris to eliminate areas that provide shade and moisture. Treat under bushes, mulched areas, and under decks and porches. Wildlife and pets that are not on flea control may access even a fenced yard and pose a continued source of new flea eggs. Many formulations of yard treatments are available at home improvement stores. Read and follow instructions on package for proper application protocol.

---

several weeks to several months to eliminate the current infestation. Make sure clients know they need to treat all pets in the household, not just the flea-allergic individual.

Some effort should be made to determine the source of the infestation and eliminate it if possible. Dogs who visit other environments (e.g. public parks, dog parks, doggie

Box 6.3 Example of a Client Handout with a Customized Flea Control Program

Flea Control Program

If you have any questions after reading this handout, please do not hesitate to call us. We want to work with you in conquering the "Florida flea" so that you and your pets will derive the maximal benefit and comfort possible. Knowing a few facts about the flea life cycle is a tremendous aid in the battle against fleas. Fleas thrive at low altitudes with humidity around 70% and in temperature ranges of 65–85°F, thus making Florida a prime flea breeding ground. Under these conditions, the flea life cycle can be completed, from the hatching of the egg to the laying of the next generation of eggs, in as little as 16 days. Adult fleas spend most of their time on your pet. After the female obtains a blood meal from your pet, she lays many eggs which fall off your pet into the surrounding environment. The eggs and immature life stages of the flea hide in furniture, bedding, carpets, cracks in flooring, and in piles of leaves or mulch. **Successful flea control involves killing adult fleas as well as preventing development of immature fleas.**

For use on your pet, we suggest the following:

1) To kill adult fleas use:
   Topical
   - Activyl® every ___ weeks.
   - Activyl Tick Plus® (dogs only) every ___ weeks.
   - Advantage® every ___ weeks.
   - Advantage II® every ___ weeks.
   - K9 Advantix® (dogs only) every ___ weeks.
   - K9 Advantix II® (dogs only) every ___ weeks.
   - Frontline Plus® every ___ weeks.
   - Vectra® every ___ weeks.
   - Vectra 3D® (dogs only) every ___ weeks.
   - Advantage Multi® every ___ weeks.
   - Revolution® every ___ weeks.
   - Seresto® Collar every ___ months.
   - Scalibor® Collar (dogs only) every ___ months.

   Oral
   - Capstar® tablets every ___ days.
   - Comfortis® tablet every ___ weeks.
   - NexGard® chewables every ___ weeks.
   - Trifexis® tablets every ___ weeks.
   Which product is best for your pet depends on multiple factors including the number of pets in the household, exposure to water, exposure to other animals, and severity of the flea allergy.

2) To prevent flea eggs from hatching, consider:
   - Program®
   - Sentinel® = Contains both Program and heartworm preventative.
   - Sentinel Spectrum® = Also controls tapeworms.

Environmental Flea Control

For the House

1) Vacuum prior to any treatment method; a vacuum with a beater bar is best.
2) Professional exterminator service
   a) These tend to be less labor intensive and work very well; a good pest control operator will work with you to combat the flea problem… ask questions. Also, let them know if you have a flea-allergic pet.
   b) If you have greater than 50% carpeting in your home, consider a service that embeds a borate-like compound into your carpets. Such companies often have a 1-year service guarantee. Good to excellent results have been obtained with these services.
   c) Other exterminator services will spray your home at regular intervals. We recommend the use of an **I**nsect **G**rowth **R**egulator (IGR) such as methoprene (Precor®) or pyriproxyfen (Nylar®). Discuss with your exterminator the time interval of treatments for your home.
3) Do-it-yourself (follow label instructions carefully):

a) Concentrate under and in furniture and where pets frequent; don't forget welcome mats!

b) We recommend using insect growth regulators such as methoprene (Precor®) or pyriproxyfen (Nylar®). If the problem is severe, consider the use of an adulticide such as permethrin, bifenthrin, fenvalerate, etc.

c) Sprays are often recommended over foggers because foggers tend to go up and come down; however, they do not always get under furniture and make it difficult to treat areas adequately.

For the Yard

1) Professional exterminators or the do-it-yourself approach may be used.

2) Adulticides such as imidacloprid, cyfluthrin, bifenthrin, etc. can be applied to the yard.

3) Concentrate under shaded areas such as porches, trees, and bushes; in areas with organic debris, around the home and where pets frequent.

4) Apply products as directed every 3–4 weeks, depending on the weather, especially rainfall.

5) Biological flea control using the natural flea predator the nematode (Steinernema carpocapsae) is another alternative.

day care, open fields) are at risk for picking up newly hatched fleas and should always be treated with flea adulticides. Stray dogs and cats, and wildlife such as opossums and raccoons, are frequent sources of flea infestations, and exclusion of these visitors from the yard is recommended. Access to areas under houses, sheds, and decks should be blocked.

Client expectations about product performance must be realistic. Many clients mistakenly think the new products repel adult fleas and therefore assume fleas have become resistant if they see any fleas on their pet after application of the product. In reality, they are seeing newly hatched adult fleas that developed from immature stages already present in the environment. They must be reminded that complete flea eradication takes time. True resistance to the modern flea control products has not been documented (Blagburn et al. 2008; Dryden 1998; Payne et al. 2001).

Proper application of topical products should be explained and ideally demonstrated. Instructions for proper administration of oral medications must be followed, for instance give with a full meal. Recommendations for environmental control measures should be explained in detail, and label directions on all environmentally applied products should be followed. Indoor environmental control efforts should concentrate on areas that are suitable for flea development and where pets spend the majority of their time, including pet bedding, upholstered furniture, and carpeting. Insect growth regulators are usually all that is needed indoors unless the infestation is severe. In severe infestations, environmental application of a flea adulticide may be beneficial. Spraying of flea adulticides outdoors is usually only necessary in severe infestations and should concentrate on shaded, protected areas suitable for flea development. Clients may prefer to have a professional exterminating service treat the environment. Be sure clients tell the exterminating service they need treatment for fleas as opposed to the usual household pests such as roaches, ants, and silverfish.

Written instructions for flea control should be provided for clients to take home and refer to later. Handouts and reputable internet sites (www.drmichaeldryden.com) are also good ways to provide clients with flea biology and life cycle information. Having a written copy of the information discussed at the appointment will help clients remember the important details of their treatment plan and will increase the chances for successful flea control.

Conclusion

FAD is one of the most common skin diseases affecting dogs and cats in many areas of the world. When left untreated, it causes severe pruritus and discomfort. Fortunately for today's pets, successful treatment of FAD can almost always be achieved. The veterinary technician plays a central role in the successful management of FAD. Recognition of clinical signs, collection of relevant historical information, and extensive client education regarding flea control can all be accomplished by the technician. Client compliance is critical, and the veterinary technician with expertise about fleas can explain proper use of flea control products and provide realistic expectations about product performance, as well as length of time to disease control. Thorough client education combined with today's highly efficacious flea control products have made successful management of the flea allergic patient more achievable than ever before.

References

Blagburn, B.L., Dryden, M.W., Payne, P.A. et al. (2008). New insights into flea resistance. *Compendium: Continuing Education for Veterinarians* 30 (Suppl. 6B): 4–6.

Burrows, A. (2009). Avermectins in dermatology. In: *Kirk's Current Veterinary Therapy XIV* (eds. J.D. Bonagura and D.C. Twedt), 390–394. St. Louis, Missouri: Saunders/Elsevier.

Dryden, M.W. (1998). Laboratory evaluations of topical flea control products. In C. Curtis (ed.), *Proceedings of the British Veterinary Dermatology Study Group*. Ware: LEO Animal Health, pp. 14–17. https://www.bvdsg.org.uk/resources/29/757/81/BVDSG_1998_BW.pdf (accessed May 2019).

Elanco (2018). Comfortis® (spinosad). www.elanco.us/products-services/dogs/comfortis (accessed May 2019).

Environmental Protection Agency (2019). Reevaluation: review of registered pesticides. http://www.epa.gov/oppsrrd1/reevaluation/pyrethroids-pyrethrins.html (accessed May 2019).

Favrot, C. (2014). Clinical presentations and specificity of feline manifestations of cutaneous allergies. In: *Veterinary Allergy* (eds. C. Noli, A.P. Foster and W. Rosenkrantz), 211–216. Chichester: Wiley.

Jacobs, D.E., Hutchinson, M.J., Stanneck, D., and Mencke, N. (2001). Accumulation and persistence of flea larvicidal activity in the immediate environment of cats treated with imidacloprid. *Medical and Veterinary Entomology* 15: 342–345.

Kennis, R. (2004). Parasiticides in dermatology. In: *Small Animal Dermatolgy Secrets* (ed. K. Campbell), 65. Philadelphia: Hanley and Belfus.

Koch, S.N., Torres, S.M.F., and Plumb, D.C. (2012). *Canine and Feline Dermatology Drug Handbook, p. 191*. Ames, IA: Wiley-Blackwell.

Kunkle, G.A. and Halliwell, R.E.W. (2003). Flea allergy and flea control. In: *BSAVA Manual of Small Animal Dermatology*, 2e (eds. C.S. Foil and A.P. Foster), 137–145. Gloucester: British Small Animal Veterinary Association.

Logas, D. (2014). Clinical presentations (of feline flea bite allergy). In: *Veterinary Allergy* (eds. C. Noli, A.P. Foster and W. Rosenkrantz), 252–254. Chichester: Wiley.

McTier, T.L., Shanks, D.J., Jernigan, A.D. et al. (2000). Evaluation of the effects of selamectin against adult and immature stages of fleas (*Ctenocephalides felis felis*) on dogs and cats. *Veterinary Parasitology* 91 (3–4): 201–212.

Mencke, N. (2000). Efficacy of advantage against natural infestations of dogs with lice: a field study from Norway. *Compendium on Continuing Education for the Practicing Veterinarian* 22 (suppl): 18.

Merck Animal Health (2012). Technical monograph: Indoxacarb, the first bioactivated flea control compound. Activyl for cats. Activyl Tick Plus for dogs. Millsboro, DE: Intervet Inc., a subsidiary of Merck & Co., Inc.

Miller, W.H., Griffin, C.E., and Campbell, K.L. (2013). *Muller & Kirk's Small Animal Dermatology*, 7e. St. Louis, Missouri: Elsevier/Mosby.

Payne, P.A., Dryden, M.W., Smith, V. et al. (2001). Effect of 0.29% w/w fipronil spray on adult flea mortality and egg production of three different cat flea, *Ctenocephalideds felis* (bouche), strains infesting cats. *Veterinary Parasitology* 102: 331–340.

Rust, M.K. and Dryden, M.W. (1997). The biology, ecology, and management of the cat flea. *Annual Review of Entomology* 42: 451–473.

Rust, M.K., Waggoner, N.C., Hinkle, C. et al. (2003). Efficacy and longevity of nitenpyram against adult cat fleas (Siphonaptera: Pulicidae). *Journal of Medical Entomology* 40 (5): 678–681.

Sousa, C.A. and Halliwell, R.E.W. (2001). The ACVD task force on canine atopic dermatitis (XI): the relationship between arthropod hypersensitivity and atopic dermatitis in the dog. *Veterinary Immunology and Immunopathology* 81: 233–237.

Webliography

Dr. Flea. www.drmichaeldryden.com (accessed May 2019).

7

Atopic Dermatitis
Amanda Friedeck

Introduction

Atopic dermatitis (AD) is the second most common allergy seen in dogs and cats and is estimated to occur in 3–15% of the population (Reedy et al. 1997). AD is defined as "a genetically predisposed, inflammatory and pruritic allergic skin disease with characteristic clinical features associated with IgE antibodies most commonly directed against environmental allergens" (Halliwell 2006). AD is often a chronic problem that can be controlled, but not cured.

Successful management of patients with AD requires thorough and complete client education. These patients often require multiple therapies to achieve an acceptable level of comfort and these therapies may need to be continued for the life of the patient. Owners who have a good understanding of AD are more likely to follow therapeutic recommendations. These owners also tend to be more observant and report problems such as secondary infections sooner to their veterinarian. This leads to better disease control and increased patient comfort.

Pathogenesis

The pathogenesis of canine AD is extremely complex and many of its details remain to be discovered; however, it is important for the veterinary technician to have a basic understanding of the disease in order to explain it to clients. AD is the result of a pro-inflammatory response of the immune system to environmental allergens. Both genetic and environmental factors are involved in the development of AD. Allergen exposure occurs via the respiratory tract, oral mucous membranes, and, most importantly for canine AD, the skin. Allergen exposure in atopic individuals results in the production of allergen-specific immunoglobulin E (IgE), as well as numerous inflammatory cytokines (intercellular chemical messengers). These cytokines cause the erythema and pruritus that are the hallmarks of AD. In addition to producing allergen-specific IgE, atopic individuals have been shown to have defects in skin barrier function that allow increased allergen absorption. The reader is encouraged to pursue more detailed discussions of the pathogenesis of AD in the references at the end of the chapter (Marsella 2010; Marsella et al. 2012; Miller et al. 2013; Noli et al. 2014; Olivry et al. 2010).

Much less is known about the pathogenesis of feline AD and evidence to confirm the hypothesis that the disease is comparable to AD in humans and dogs is lacking; therefore, feline atopic-like disease (ALD) or feline non-flea, non-food hypersensitivity dermatitis are considered more correct names for this disease in cats (Favrot 2014; Hobi et al. 2011).

Small Animal Dermatology for Technicians and Nurses, First Edition. Edited by Kim Horne, Marcia Schwassmann and Dawn Logas.
© 2020 John Wiley & Sons, Inc. Published 2020 by John Wiley & Sons, Inc.

Clinical Features (Canine)

Numerous studies have reported a wide variety of breed predispositions for AD. Local variations in breed popularity and genetic variation within breeds from different geographical locations probably account for many of these differences. Breeds listed as predisposed in multiple studies were boxers, bulldogs, German shepherd dogs, golden retrievers, Labrador retrievers, and West Highland white terriers (Favrot 2014). The hereditary basis of canine AD is well documented, but details of the complex interplay between the many genes involved remain the subject of active research. No consistent sex predilection for AD has been observed (Griffin and DeBoer 2001).

The signs of AD typically begin between six months and three years of age (Griffin and DeBoer 2001). It is rare to diagnose dogs older than seven years with AD (Griffin and DeBoer 2001), unless they have moved from a geographical area with low allergen loads to an area with higher allergen loads. Signs may be seasonal, non-seasonal (year round), or non-seasonal with seasonal exacerbations. Up to 75% of patients start out with seasonal symptoms, but most eventually become non-seasonal (Griffin and DeBoer 2001). One would expect a higher incidence of non-seasonal AD in warmer areas with year-round growing seasons.

The primary clinical sign of canine AD is pruritus (Favrot 2014) and this is often the client's presenting complaint. Many patients will have minimal cutaneous changes early in the disease (Favrot 2014; Miller et al. 2013). Erythema, erythematous macules, or small erythematous papules may be present (Favrot 2014; Miller et al. 2013; Figures 7.1 and 7.2). As AD progresses, more cutaneous changes that reflect the chronic self-trauma and secondary infections that occur will be seen. Papules, pustules, epidermal collarettes, alopecia, crusts, excoriations, lichenification, hyperpigmentation, salivary staining, and seborrhea oleosa may be seen (Favrot 2014; Miller et al. 2013; Figures 7.3–7.10). The typical

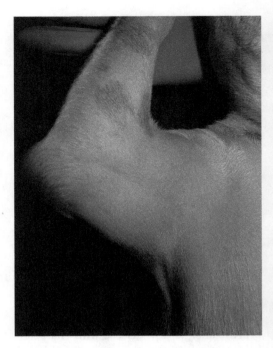

Figure 7.1 Canine with mild atopic dermatitis presenting with clinical signs of papules on the medial aspect of the right elbow.

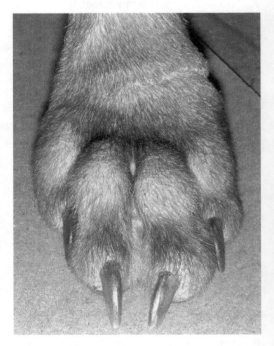

Figure 7.2 Canine with atopic dermatitis presenting with clinical sign of erythema and alopecia on the dorsal aspect of the paw.

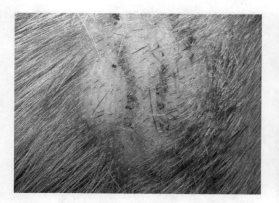

Figure 7.3 Canine patient showing excoriations.

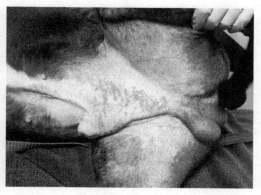

Figure 7.6 Canine with moderate atopic dermatitis presenting with partial to complete alopecia on the ventrum extending down both rear medial thighs, including the caudal aspect of both pelvic limbs. A papular rash is present, with moderate erythema and linear excoriations.

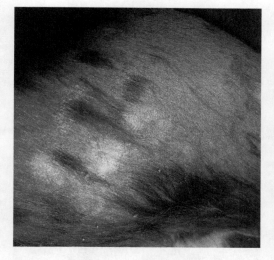

Figure 7.4 Canine with mild atopic dermatitis showing clinical sign of collarettes on the left lateral thorax.

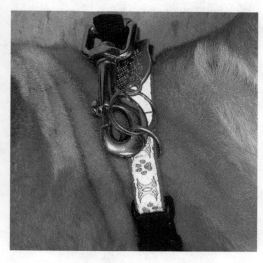

Figure 7.7 Canine with moderate atopic dermatitis with severe erythema on ventral surface of the neck.

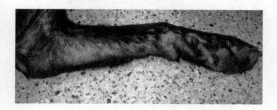

Figure 7.5 Canine with mild to moderate atopic dermatitis with diffuse partial to complete alopecia extending along the medial aspect of the left thoracic limb into the axilla, with erythema, mild scale, and a papular rash.

distribution pattern for AD includes the muzzle, periocular area, ear pinnae, ventrum (axillae, abdomen, inguinal area), flexural surface of elbows, and paws (Favrot 2014; Miller et al. 2013; Figures 7.11–7.14). One, several, or all of these areas may be affected (Favrot 2014; Griffin and DeBoer 2001).

Otitis externa is often associated with AD, with one study reporting an 86% rate of otitis externa in AD patients (Griffin and DeBoer 2001).

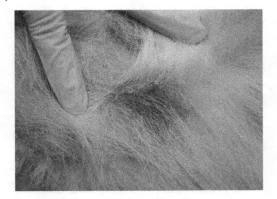

Figure 7.8 Canine with moderate atopic dermatitis with large epidermal collarettes, partial alopecia, and mild lichenification.

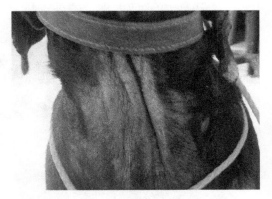

Figure 7.9 Canine patient with lichenification on ventral neck.

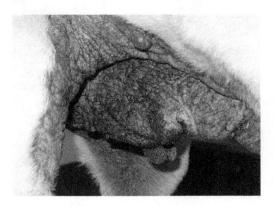

Figure 7.10 Canine with chronic atopic dermatitis presenting with severe lichenification and hyperpigmentation of the flank, ventrum, and medial aspects of the pelvic limbs. Moderate amounts of tightly adhered crust with mild ulcerations were also noted.

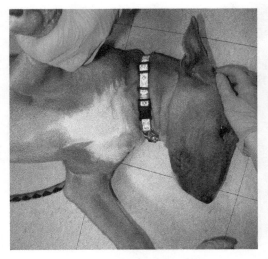

Figure 7.11 Canine with severe erythema on the ventral surface of the neck and axilla extending down to the medial surface of the thoracic limbs. Erythema can also be seen on the lateral aspect of the muzzle and concave pinna.

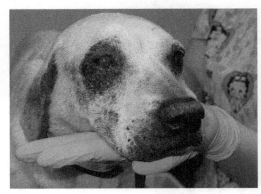

Figure 7.12 Canine with chronic atopic dermatitis with severe hyperpigmentation bilaterally in the periocular region, with tightly adhered crust and purulent ocular discharge. Mild hyperkeratosis is noted on the bridge of the nose. Moderate to severe erythema can be seen on the concave and convex surfaces of the pinna, with lacy hyperpigmentation. The muzzle is hyperpigmented, with tightly adhered crust on the lateral aspect.

Other manifestations of AD may include acute moist dermatitis, acral pruritic nodules, and acral lick granulomas (Miller et al. 2013; Figures 7.15 and 7.16). Non-cutaneous signs of AD are uncommonly reported. These include rhinitis, sneezing, and conjunctivitis. The true

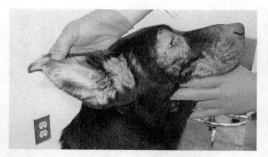

Figure 7.13 Canine with moderate atopic dermatitis, with partial to complete alopecia of the muzzle, periaural, and periocular regions. Partial alopecia is also noted on the concave surface of the pinna, as well as mild scale and tightly adhered crust on the medial aspect of the face.

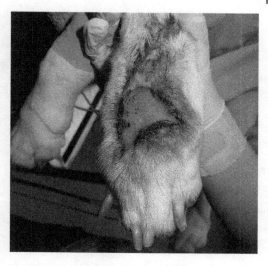

Figure 7.15 Acral lick lesion of the right carpus of a canine. A large ulcerative thickened lesion with scarring and salivary staining of the hair surrounding the lesion.

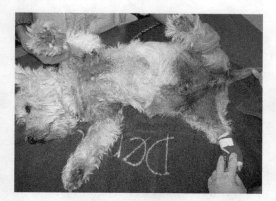

Figure 7.14 Canine with chronic untreated atopic dermatitis. Complete alopecia in the axilla and groin, with partial alopecia extending down all four limbs and ventral surface of the tail. The axilla is moist, with crusting on the leading margins of the ulcers and mild hyperpigmentation. The ventrum has severe hyperpigmentation and lichenification, with ulcerative, moist areas on the lower medial thighs, cranial to the prepuce and the perineal region.

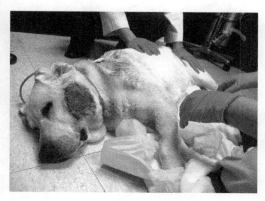

Figure 7.16 Acute moist dermatitis of a canine on the left cheek and dorsal aspect of the left shoulder. A large purulent ulcerated area, with tightly adhered crust surrounding the lesion. Typically is covered in a tightly adhered crust of blood, hair, and purulent material.

incidence of non-cutaneous signs of AD remains unknown (Griffin and DeBoer 2001). AD can occur together with other allergies such as flea allergy and food allergy, thus it is important to control concurrent allergies in these patients.

Clinical Features (Feline)

Familial and breed predispositions for feline ALD have been seen, but are less well documented than in dogs. Clinical signs often begin before three years of age (Favrot 2014; Miller et al. 2013). Pruritus is a consistent feature of the disease and many owners will report excessive grooming, licking, or scratching. Some cats, however, will only over-groom in private and these owners may insist their pet is not pruritic. A trichogram demonstrating blunted ends of hair shafts can confirm self-induced alopecia in these cases (Figure 7.17). Cats with ALD can present with a variety of clinical signs, including miliary dermatitis, head and neck pruritus, bilaterally symmetric self-induced alopecia, and eosinophilic granuloma complex lesions (Favrot 2014; Hobi et al. 2011; Figures 7.18–7.20). The head, face, ears, abdomen, neck, and hind limbs are most commonly affected (Hobi et al. 2011; Figures 7.21–7.23). Non-dermatological signs sometimes reported in association with feline ALD include sneezing, conjunctivitis, and feline asthma.

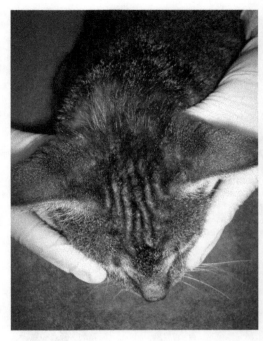

Figure 7.19 Head and neck pruritus of a feline. Mild to moderate erythema, with partial to sparse alopecia and a barbered feel to the coat. Small, tightly adhered crusts are noted on the head and neck.

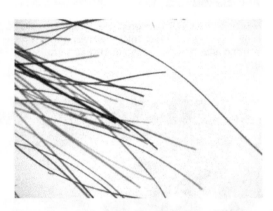

Figure 7.17 Trichogram showing barbered hairs seen at 5x magnification. Note the normal structure to the hair, but the ends are blunted, indicating broken hairs from self-induced over-grooming.

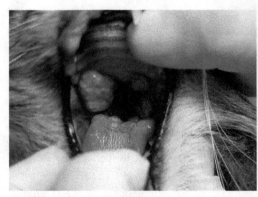

Figure 7.20 Eosinophilic granuloma complex in a feline with atopic dermatitis. Note the rodent ulcer on the upper right lip.

Diagnostic Tests

The diagnosis of AD or ALD is a clinical one and is based on history, clinical signs, and ruling out other causes of pruritic skin disease (Miller et al. 2013). Because history is

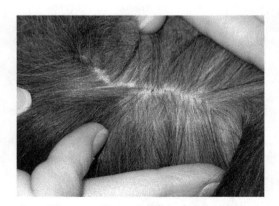

Figure 7.18 Miliary dermatitis of the feline. Very small crusts along the dorsum.

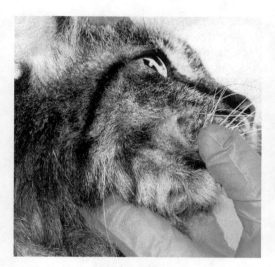

Figure 7.21 Ulcerative excoriations on the periaural and lateral aspects of the face of a feline.

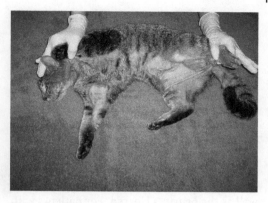

Figure 7.23 Self-induced alopecia in a feline with atopic dermatitis. Barbered hair with partial to complete alopecia in the axilla extending down the thoracic limbs, and on the ventrum extending down the pelvic limbs to encompass the cranial aspect of the knee and the caudal aspect of the thigh. The perineal region and ventral surface of the tail are also involved. Diffuse moderate to severe erythema is noted within the alopecic areas and on the face. Crust, excoriations, and partial alopecia are noted on the head, cheeks, and neck areas. Some partial alopecia can be seen on the medial aspect of the tarsus.

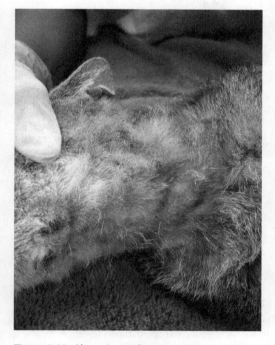

Figure 7.22 Alopecia, erythema, and crusts on the ventral neck of a feline.

so important to making the diagnosis, the veterinary technician should be skilled at obtaining a complete and accurate history from the owner.

Clients presenting pets for skin and ear problems should always be asked if their pet is pruritic. When asking about pruritus, it is important to realize that clients may not understand that licking, chewing, and rubbing are all manifestations of pruritus, not just scratching. It can be helpful to have clients grade their pet's pruritus, either using a scale of 0–10 with 0 representing no pruritus and 10 representing non-stop, severe pruritus, or using the visual analog scale described in Chapter 1. These scales can also be used to evaluate the effectiveness of therapy at recheck visits. The pruritus should be characterized as seasonal, year round, or year round with seasonal exacerbations. If seasonality is present, the time of year the patient is affected should be noted. It is also important to document which areas of the body are pruritic.

The age of the patient at the onset of the problem should be noted, as well as whether the onset was gradual or sudden. If the problem is seasonal, inquiring when the symptoms typically start and end is important. The client should be asked if the problem is stable or if it is worsening or changing in nature. Clients should be asked to describe the lesions that are present and they should also be asked if pruritus is noted prior to the development of lesions. Most dogs with AD will show pruritus before lesions develop.

Clients should be asked to list previous treatments and responses to those treatments. If response was noted, the client should be asked specifically if the lesions as well as the pruritus cleared. For patients with a long history, it may be helpful to have clients bring to their appointment a list of current and previous medications, both systemic and topical. Clients should be asked if they bathe their pet and, if so, how often and which shampoo they use. The presence of other affected pets or people in the household should be documented and can be helpful in ruling out some of the other infectious causes of pruritus, such as scabies. All clients should be asked about flea control measures being used. One or two open-ended questions concerning other abnormalities may be helpful in eliciting the presence of signs the client may not realize are significant.

Questions about the pet's environment are also important. Clients should be asked if pets spend most of their time indoors or out-

doors. Any environmental changes related to the dermatological condition should also be documented. Having a questionnaire that clients can fill out prior to their appointment can make gathering all pertinent historical information easier. See Chapter 1 for an example of a client questionnaire.

A very important part of the diagnosis of AD and ALD is ruling out other causes of pruritic dermatitis. These other causes of pruritus include parasitic diseases such as scabies and demodicosis, secondary bacterial and yeast infections, and other allergic conditions such as flea allergy dermatitis and food allergy (DeBoer and Hillier 2001a; Miller et al. 2013).

It must be made clear that there is no diagnostic test that tells you if a patient's current signs are due to flea allergy, food allergy, or AD. Flea allergy is ruled out with intensive flea control and food allergy is ruled out with an elimination diet trial. Some patients may have more than one type of allergic condition, which can make the diagnostic process quite complex. If the history and clinical signs fit, and all other pruritic diseases have been ruled out or controlled, then the diagnosis of AD or ALD can be made. "Allergy testing," either by intradermal testing (Box 7.1 and Figure 7.24) or measurement of serum IgE levels (Box 7.2), is a therapeutic

---

Box 7.1 Intradermal Allergy Testing Information

Intradermal testing (IDT) is the most accepted form of "allergy" testing. It consists of the intradermal injection of small volumes of allergens, typically a series of grass pollens, weed pollens, tree pollens, house dust mites, insects, molds, and epidermals. Saline is used for the negative control and histamine is used as the positive control. The resulting wheal is then subjectively graded based on size, degree of erythema, and turgidity. The reactions are usually graded as 0–4, with 0 representing no reaction, and 4 being a reaction equal to that of the histamine. Some dermatologists prefer to use measurement of wheal diameters as a way of grading the reactions.

IDT is usually done by a dermatologist, since a certain amount of expertise is required to read the test and frequent testing must be performed to justify the expense of keeping a panel of in-date allergens. IDT is usually done with the patient under sedation and obtaining valid test results may require the discontinuation of certain medications, e.g. antihistamines and glucocorticoids, for a specified period of time before the test. Recommended drug withdrawal times vary, so consultation with the dermatologist who will perform the test is recommended.

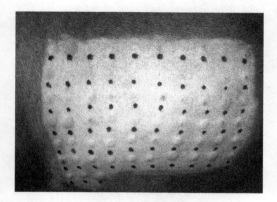

Figure 7.24 Intradermal allergy test results, canine patient.

Box 7.2 Serum Allergy Testing Information

Serum "allergy" testing measures levels of allergen-specific IgE, most often using either radioallergosorbent (RAST) or enzyme-linked immunosorbent assay (ELISA) techniques. It has traditionally been recommended when intradermal testing (IDT) is not possible, although some dermatologists recommend a combination of IDT and serum testing. Many laboratories offer serum "allergy" testing for foods. This is not an accurate method of determining food allergies and is not recommended. Serum testing is not as widely accepted as IDT due to the wide range of specificity and sensitivity for these tests that is reported in the literature (Deboer and Hillier 2001b). Care should also be taken when choosing a laboratory to perform serum "allergy" testing, as standardization and quality control measures are determined by each individual laboratory and results can vary widely between laboratories (Plant et al. 2014; Deboer and Hillier 2001b).

---

tool used to identify individual allergens for avoidance or for inclusion in allergen-specific immunotherapy (ASIT). Avoidance is often impractical, so the client should understand that the primary goal of "allergy testing" is to determine which allergens to include in ASIT.

Treatment

Treatment of AD or ALD requires a multimodal approach consisting of a combination of topical and systemic therapies. The goal is to maximize clinical improvement while minimizing adverse effects of therapy. Treatment will vary depending on the duration and severity of clinical signs, as well as the patient's tolerance of therapies and the capabilities of the owner. Therapy is directed at minimizing allergen exposure (e.g. frequent bathing to remove allergens from the skin, improving skin barrier function), decreasing the immune system's inflammatory reaction to allergen exposure (drug therapy or ASIT), controlling secondary infections (e.g. bacterial pyoderma and yeast), and controlling any concurrent allergies (e.g. flea and/or food allergy; Olivry and Sousa 2001a; Miller et al. 2013). Treatments differ in their ease of use, cost, effectiveness, and side-effect profile.

Topical therapy is an integral part of the treatment of canine AD and can decrease the need for systemic therapy. Whole body shampoos and conditioners are utilized for generalized pruritus, while topical creams, ointments, and sprays may be useful for more localized pruritus. Topical therapy such as bathing is used less frequently in cats, but can be effective if accepted by the patient.

Bathing removes surface debris, microorganisms, and allergens from the skin surface (Miller et al. 2013). Hypoallergenic and moisturizing shampoos are generally recommended for dogs with AD, since they often need frequent bathing. Antimicrobial shampoos may be used to help prevent or control secondary bacterial and yeast infections on the skin. Shampoo ingredients with good antibacterial activity include benzoyl peroxide, chlorhexidine, and ethyl lactate. Antifungal agents found in shampoos include miconazole, ketoconazole, chlorhexidine, selenium sulfide, and sulfur (Miller et al. 2013). Antipruritic shampoos can also be a useful adjunct therapy for AD. Antipruritic agents include colloidal oatmeal, pramoxine (a topical anesthetic), diphenhydramine (an antihistamine), and hydrocortisone (Miller et al. 2013). A newer class of shampoos, sprays, and pour-ons designed to repair the defective skin barrier function associated with AD has recently been developed. These products may contain phytosphingosine, ceramides, or fatty acids. Large, blinded, placebo-controlled clinical trials to evaluate the efficacy of these products have not yet been completed. Conditioners and leave-on rinses with moisturizing, antipruritic, and antimicrobial properties are also available and may provide some added benefit because they are allowed to remain on the skin. Whichever product is recommended, providing the client with information and tips on how to properly bathe their pet is helpful (Box 7.3).

Many products for localized application are available as sprays, creams, lotions, gels, and wipes. These products may contain antibacterial, antifungal, antipruritic, and anti-inflammatory agents.

Most AD/ALD patients will require some form of systemic therapy in addition to their topical therapy. Mild cases may respond to antihistamines and fatty acid supplementation, while more severe cases may require

---

Box 7.3 Bathing Tips to Share with Clients

Clients should initially receive detailed instructions on how to properly bathe their dog. Dogs may accept being bathed in a tub more easily if they are rewarded with treats and if non-skid bath mats are utilized. Cool to lukewarm water should be used to thoroughly wet the coat. Shampoo can be squirted onto the owner's hands and then gently rubbed into the coat. Gentle massage should be used to promote lather formation, but vigorous scrubbing (especially against the direction of hair growth) should be avoided, as this can lead to traumatic folliculitis in short-coated dogs. Clients should be cautioned not to apply a thick stream of shampoo to the animal's dorsal midline and attempt to spread the shampoo outward from there, as this results in too much shampoo in a focal area that may be difficult to rinse off completely. All areas of the body should be washed, including the feet and face. Care should be taken to avoid getting shampoo into the eyes. If this does happen, gently rinse immediately with plenty of water.

Clients should be encouraged to use a clock or other timer to ensure adequate contact time is achieved (usually at least 10 minutes). Shampoo should be applied to the more severely affected area first to facilitate longer contact times. The timer should be started once the entire pet is lathered. If pets are being bathed outdoors, they can go for a walk while the shampoo is soaking. Owners should also be advised that many medicated shampoos do not lather well. Animals that are particularly dirty can be washed with a cleansing shampoo first before using the medicated shampoo. Some dogs with long, thick coats will benefit from having the coat clipped shorter to facilitate contact of shampoo with the skin. This also may decrease the amount of shampoo that is used, as well as drying time.

Thorough rinsing is extremely important, as shampoo residue can cause irritation. Animals with thick coats may require more time for rinsing than for shampooing. Particular attention should be paid to the axillae, inguinal area, caudal thighs, and feet to ensure all shampoo has been removed. Bath time is also a good time for ear cleaning and application of a drying ear rinse after a bath can ensure water does not remain in the ear canals. Short-coated dogs can be toweled almost dry and then be allowed to air dry as long as they do not become chilled. Longer-coated dogs may need to be blow dried and brushed. Care should be taken to use the cooler settings on a blow dryer to avoid irritating sensitive skin. The frequency of bathing recommended will vary depending on the severity of the skin condition, but most dogs with atopic dermatitis will benefit from baths at least once every 1–2 weeks.

glucocorticoids, cyclosporine, oclacitinib (dogs only), or CYTOPOINT® (canine monoclonal antibodies to interleukin-31). Despite lack of conclusive evidence for their benefit, antihistamines such as diphenhydramine, hydroxyzine, chlorpheniramine, loratadine, and cetirizine are commonly prescribed (DeBoer and Griffin 2001; Olivry et al. 2010). Individual patient response to antihistamines varies considerably, so several different options may need to be tried. Antihistamines have limited effectiveness, so are best used for patients with mild pruritus. Their most common side effect is sedation (DeBoer and Griffin 2001). Clients must take care not to give their pets over-the-counter products that contain antihistamines together with decongestants or pain relievers, as these other drugs may be toxic at doses appropriate for humans.

Essential fatty acid supplementation may reduce pruritus in some dogs with AD (Olivry et al. 2010; Miller et al. 2013). Essential fatty acids decrease the production of inflammatory mediators and may improve the barrier function of the skin (Miller et al. 2013). Increased amounts of fatty acids can be incorporated into the diet or can be given separately in capsule or liquid form, and it may take several months to see a response.

Glucocorticoids are very effective at quickly reducing pruritus, but they should be used sparingly due to their potential for adverse effects. Also because of these adverse effects, short-acting oral glucocorticoids are usually preferred over long-acting injectable formulations. Acute side effects include polyuria, polydipsia, polyphagia, and panting. These side effects resolve when the glucocorticoid therapy is discontinued (Olivry and Sousa 2001b). More chronic use may be associated with liver damage, thin skin, hair loss, diabetes mellitus, increased susceptibility to urinary tract infections, increased susceptibility to other infections, obesity, and, less often, gastrointestinal ulceration, pulmonary thromboembolism, pancreatitis, and calcinosis cutis (Miller et al. 2013). Monitoring of patients on chronic glucocorticoid therapy should include periodic physical examinations, chemistry panels, urinalyses, and urine cultures (Miller et al. 2013).

Cyclosporine A is an immunosuppressive drug that has shown good efficacy for the treatment of AD in dogs (DeBoer 2014; Miller et al. 2013; Olivry et al. 2010). It is not a glucocorticoid and therefore avoids the adverse effects associated with glucocorticoid use. The most common adverse effect of cyclosporine is gastrointestinal upset. Patients may show decreased appetite, vomiting, or diarrhea. Temporarily stopping the drug, giving the drug with food, freezing the capsule, temporarily decreasing the drug dosage, giving half the dose twice a day, or giving anti-vomiting medication may decrease gastrointestinal upset (Miller et al. 2013). Other reported side effects include hirsutism, bacterial skin infection, gingival hyperplasia, and papillomatosis (Miller et al. 2013; Figures 7.25 and 7.26). Chronic cyclosporine therapy may predispose to urinary tract infections, so urinalyses and urine cultures should be monitored periodically (Peterson et al. 2011). The microemulsion form of cyclosporine (Atopica®, Elanco US Inc, Greenfield, IN, USA) has better absorption than the non-modified form (Sandimmune®, Novartis) and the two cannot be used interchangeably. The absorption of human generic formulations of modified cyclosporine in dogs varies, so use of the veterinary brand-name product is recommended (Miller et al. 2013). Cyclosporine does interact with a number of other drugs, so a detailed patient medication history should be obtained from the client before starting cyclosporine therapy (Koch et al. 2012; Plumb 2011). Concurrent administration of ketoconazole and cyclosporine can increase blood levels of cyclosporine and this interaction is sometimes used to decrease the required dose of cyclosporine, thereby reducing the cost of therapy (Miller et al. 2013).

Oclacitinib (Apoquel®, Zoetis, Parsippany, NJ) is the newest non-steroidal drug

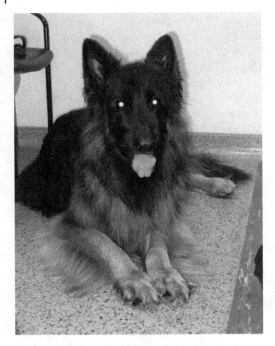

Figure 7.25 Hirsutism of a German shepherd dog from cyclosporine administration. Note the excessive hair growth on his chest and limbs.

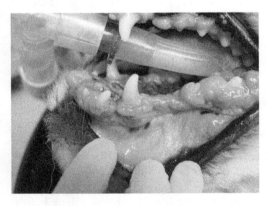

Figure 7.26 Severe gingival hyperplasia in a canine on cyclosporine.

approved for the treatment of canine AD. It is a Janus Kinase (JAK) inhibitor that decreases production of the cytokines responsible for the itch sensation and inflammation. Oclacitinib typically provides a rapid decrease in pruritus with minimal adverse effects (Cosgrove et al. 2013; DeBoer 2014).

It is approved for use in dogs greater than 12 months of age, but has a label warning that the drug "may increase susceptibility to infection, including demodicosis, and may exacerbate neoplastic conditions" (Zoetis 2016).

Zoetis has also recently developed a monoclonal antibody to interleukin-31, the cytokine responsible for causing the itch sensation in dogs with AD. These antibodies bind to and neutralize interleukin-31. They are administered as a subcutaneous injection that can provide relief from itching for one to two months. Preliminary data indicates this product is very safe and effective, with no known contraindications (Zoetis n.d.).

ASIT is one of the best long-term treatment options for AD and ALD. The patient receives subcutaneous injections of an individualized mixture of allergen extracts on a regular basis. This controlled exposure decreases the immune system's reactivity to the allergens, thereby decreasing the patient's clinical signs. The primary advantage of immunotherapy is its lack of adverse effects associated with long-term use. Results of numerous studies, although open and uncontrolled, have shown improvements of 50% or more in 50–100% of patients evaluated (Griffin and Hillier 2001). ASIT may require several months before improvement is seen, so these patients will need symptomatic therapy during that time period. Response to ASIT can be complete or partial and clients must be made aware of this fact (Mueller 2014). Patients who respond to ASIT may need to continue injections indefinitely (Miller et al. 2013) or, if response to therapy is complete, they may consider stopping injections after three years (Griffin and Hillier 2001). There is currently insufficient data from controlled studies in dogs to make more specific recommendations regarding the required length of ASIT. Patients can have adverse reactions to the injections, which may include localized erythema and swelling, a more generalized increase in pruritus, and very rarely angioedema, urticaria, or anaphylaxis (Mueller 2014; Miller et al. 2013). Unlike in humans, laryngeal edema is not a common manifestation of anaphylaxis in dogs. Sudden onset of vomiting, diarrhea, and circulatory system collapse that manifests as weakness, collapse, and pale mucous membranes are more typical signs of anaphylaxis in dogs (Miller et al. 2013).

Each patient's allergens of importance can be identified by intradermal testing or measurement of allergen-specific IgE levels in serum. Allergens to be included in the treatment set are selected based on the patient's history, the strength of the positive reaction on the allergy test, and the prevalence of the allergen in the patient's environment. The number of allergens included in a treatment set has traditionally been 10–12; however, some sets may contain many more allergens. Various protocols for injection schedules are used, with the goal of maintenance administration every one to three weeks (Koch et al. 2012). The amount of allergen injected as well as the interval between injections may need to be adjusted based on each individual patient's response to immunotherapy. The client can usually be taught to administer the subcutaneous injections at home (Figures 7.27 and 7.28). ASIT is prescribed

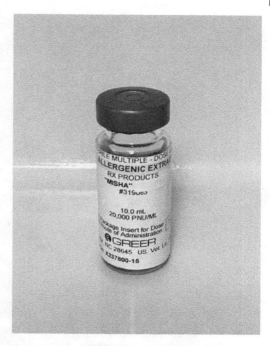

Figure 7.28 Injectable immunotherapy, prepared commercially. *Source:* Photo by Jamie Fischer, courtesy of the University of Minnesota, College of Veterinary Medicine.

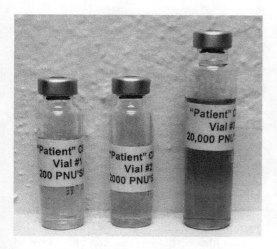

Figure 7.27 Injectable immunotherapy starter set, prepared in-house. Three vials each with a different concentration (200 PNU (protein nitrogen units), 2,000 PNU, and 20,000 PNU). Treatment is started with the lowest concentration, progressing to the last vial at the maintenance concentration.

most often by veterinary dermatologists due to the time and expertise required for management of this treatment (Miller et al. 2013).

Sublingual/intraoral administration of ASIT has recently become available for use in dogs (Figures 7.29 and 7.30). A multicenter open study demonstrated good efficacy equivalent to injectable immunotherapy (DeBoer and Morris 2012); however, blinded, placebo-controlled studies are needed to confirm this finding. This treatment option may be preferred by clients who are not comfortable giving injections, but they must be made aware that this therapy requires at least once-daily administration and several protocols recommend twice-daily dosing (Heska n.d.; Stallergenes Greer 2018). The immunotherapy mixture must be administered into the oral cavity (not put in food or treats), and the dog should not eat or drink for 10 minutes prior to or after treatment (Heska n.d.; Stallergenes Greer 2018).

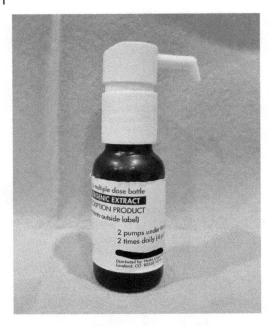

Figure 7.29 Sublingual immunotherapy administration vial, prepared commercially. The curved tip allows for easy administration into the oral cavity. Two pumps of allergy drops under the tongue are recommended to be given twice daily, every day.

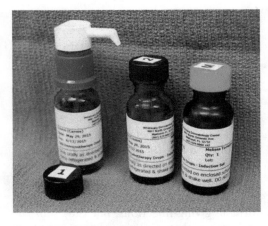

Figure 7.30 Sublingual immunotherapy starter set, prepared in-house. Treatment is started with the lowest concentration, progressing to the last vial at the maintenance concentration.

Allergen avoidance may be helpful as adjunct therapy in certain cases (Morris 2014). Patients with house dust mite allergies may benefit from house dust mite control measures. Replacing carpeting with hard-surface flooring and replacing upholstered furniture with leather furniture may decrease house dust mite burdens in the environment. Dust mite-impermeable mattress covers may be beneficial for pets that sleep with their owners. Pet bedding should also have dust mite-impermeable covers if the entire bed cannot be washed. If possible, once-weekly washing of bedding in hot water is recommended. Keeping pets out of dusty areas such as closets, under beds, and out of rooms being vacuumed can also be beneficial. Products that denature mite allergens and kill dust mites in carpeting are also available.

If pets have mold allergies, decreasing indoor mold exposure may be helpful, for example keeping pets out of moldy basements or areas with water damage. Outdoor mold avoidance can be more difficult, especially in warm, humid climates. Pollen avoidance is much more challenging. Bathing can remove pollens from the skin surface and some pets benefit from bathing after being outside or going swimming. Grass pollen–allergic patients may benefit from avoiding contact with grass.

Client Education

The successful management of AD requires the collaborative effort of the veterinary staff and the owner of the atopic patient. The veterinary technician is ideally placed to deliver much of the information and support clients will need in order to care for their atopic pets. These patients often require intensive follow-up, both with recheck appointments and phone call communication, and it can take time to find the best combination of topical and systemic therapies for each patient. Clients must understand that AD is often a lifelong disease that can be controlled but not cured. They must realize that disease flare-ups will occur and that the goal of therapy is to minimize the frequency and severity of these flare-ups. It is sometimes helpful to compare the pet with AD to a person with allergic rhinitis or asthma. This makes it easier for the client to grasp the chronic nature of the condition. The more the client understands about AD, the less frustration they will experience in dealing with the disease. Clients must also be made aware that treatment for severe AD can be expensive, and veterinary staff must be sure the therapy recommended fits into the client's budget and time constraints.

The multifaceted nature of therapy for AD should be explained to clients. They must understand that AD patients with concurrent flea bite allergy need constant, year-round (depending on geographical location) flea control. AD patients with concurrent food allergies must avoid the offending food allergens. Bacterial and yeast infections that occur secondary to AD flare-ups must be treated and hopefully prevented with maintenance topical antimicrobial therapy. Allergen avoidance should be practiced whenever possible. Bathing immediately after inadvertent pollen exposure may decrease percutaneous allergen absorption and the severity of the flare-up.

The amount of information clients need to manage AD patients can be overwhelming, so written instructions are very important. It can be helpful to have handouts or recommended websites for clients who want additional disease information and general therapeutic recommendations. Every client should also go home with a written list of instructions and medications from each appointment. The technician should review this list with the owner to ensure they understand all instructions and are able to comply with the veterinarian's recommendations. Possible side effects of medications should be briefly reviewed and clients should be encouraged to call the office if they have any questions or if the pet is having any problems with the medications.

Clients should be encouraged to be as proactive as possible when dealing with AD, because the disease is more responsive to therapy before chronic skin changes occur. They should be encouraged to make recommended recheck appointments and to contact the office if the pet is having flare-ups. Regular follow-up phone calls can be helpful for identifying patients who are having problems.

Conclusion

The veterinary staff must remember that every patient is an individual and therapy must be tailored to each patient and client. Good listening skills, patience, empathy, and good communication are essential skills for the veterinary technician when dealing with AD patients and their owners. Successful management of AD can be time consuming as well as very rewarding. The goal is to make each patient as comfortable as possible, with therapy that is the most effective with the fewest side effects.

References

Cosgrove, S.B., Wren, J.A., Cleaver, D.M. et al. (2013). A blinded, randomized, placebo-controlled trial of the efficacy and safety of the Janus kinase inhibitor oclacitinib (Apoquel®) in client-owned dogs with atopic dermatitis. *Veterinary Dermatology* 24: 587–e142. https://doi.org/10.1111/vde.12088.

DeBoer, D.J. and Griffin, C.E. (2001). The ACVD Task Force on Canine Atopic Dermatitis (XXI): antihistamine pharmacotherapy. *Veterinary Immunology and Immunopathology* 81: 324–329.

DeBoer, D.J. and Hillier, A. (2001a). The ACVD Task Force on Canine Atopic Dermatitis (XV); fundamental concepts in clinical diagnosis. *Veterinary Immunology and Immunopathology* 81: 271–276.

DeBoer, D.J. and Hillier, A. (2001b). The ACVD Task Force on Canine Atopic Dermatitis (XVI): laboratory evaluation of dogs with atopic dermatitis with serum-based "allergy" tests. *Veterinary Immunology and Immunopathology* 81: 277–287.

DeBoer, D. and Morris, M. (2012). Multicentre open trial demonstrates efficacy of sublingual immunotherapy in canine atopic dermatitis (abst.). *Vet Dermatol* 23 (Suppl 1): 65.

DeBoer, D.J. (2014). Guidelines for symptomatic medical treatment of canine atopic dermatitis. In: *Veterinary Allergy* (eds. C. Noli, A. Foster and W. Rosenkrantz), 90–95. Chichester: Wiley Blackwell.

Favrot, C. (2014). Clinical presentations and specificity of feline manifestations of cutaneous allergies. In: *Veterinary Allergy* (eds. C. Noli, A. Foster and W. Rosenkrantz), 211–216. Chichester: Wiley Blackwell.

Griffin, C.E. and DeBoer, D.J. (2001). The ACVD Task Force on Canine Atopic Dermatitis (XIV): clinical manifestations of canine atopic dermatitis. *Veterinary Immunology and Immunopathology* 81: 255–269.

Griffin, C.E. and Hillier, A. (2001). The ACVD Task Force on Canine Atopic Dermatitis (XXIV): allergen-specific immunotherapy. *Veterinary Immunology and Immunopathology* 81: 363–383.

Halliwell, R. (2006). Revised nomenclature for veterinary allergy. *Veterinary Immunology and Immunopathology* 114 (3–4): 207–208.

Heska (n.d.) ALLERCEPT® therapy drops. http://www.heska.com/Products/ALLERCEPT/Allercept-Drops.aspx (accessed May 2015).

Hobi, S., Linek, M., Marignac, G. et al. (2011). Clinical characteristics and causes of pruritus in cats: a multicentre study on feline hypersensitivity-associated dermatoses. *Veterinary Dermatology* 22: 406–413.

Koch, S.N., Torres, S.M.F., and Plumb, D.C. (2012). *Canine and Feline Dermatology Drug Handbook*, 1e. Ames, IA: Wiley Blackwell.

Marsella, R. (2010). Canine atopic dermatitis: what's new? Comp Cont Educ Vet., Feb.: E1–E4. http://vetfolio-vetstreet.s3.amazonaws.com/mmah/07/e9db03ba26460490b370f052bc5511/filePV0210_Marsella_Derm.pdf (accessed May 2019).

Marsella, R., Sousa, C.A., Gonzales, A.J., and Fadok, V.A. (2012). Current understanding of the pathophysiologic mechanisms of canine atopic dermatitis. *Journal of the American Veterinary Medical Association* 241 (2): 194–207.

Miller, W.H., Griffin, C.E., and Campbell, K.L. (2013). *Muller and Kirk's Small Animal Dermatology*, 7e. St. Louis, Missouri: Elsevier.

Morris, D.O. (2014). Allergen avoidance. In: *Veterinary Allergy* (eds. C. Noli, A.P. Foster and W. Rosenkrantz), 78–85. Chichester: Wiley.

Mueller, R.S. (2014). Allergen-specific immunotherapy. In: *Veterinary Allergy* (eds. C. Noli, A.P. Foster and W. Rosenkrantz), 86–90. Chichester: Wiley.

Noli, C., Foster, A., and Rosenkrantz, W. (eds.) (2014). *Veterinary Allergy*. Chichester: Wiley.

Olivry, T. and Sousa, C.A. (2001a). The ACVD Task Force on Canine Atopic Dermatitis (XIX): general principles of therapy. *Veterinary Immunology and Immunopathology* 81: 311–316.

Olivry, T. and Sousa, C.A. (2001b). The ACVD Task Force on Canine Atopic Dermatitis (XX): glucocorticoid pharmacotherapy. *Veterinary Immunology and Immunopathology* 81: 317–322.

Olivry, T., DeBoer, D.J., Favrot, C. et al. (2010). Treatment of Canine Atopic Dermatitis: 2010 clinical practice guidelines from the International Task Force on canine Atopic Dermatitis. *Veterinary Dermatology* (21): 233–248.

Peterson, A., Torres, S., and Rendahl, A. (2011). Frequency of urinary tract infection in dogs treated with oral ciclosporin: a retrospective study of 87 cases. *Veterinary Dermatology* 22 (3): 291–292.

Plant, J.D., Neradelik, M.B., Polissar, M.L. et al. (2014). Agreement between allergen-specific IgE assays and ensuing immunotherapy recommendations from four commercial laboratories in the USA. *Veterinary Dermatology* 25 (1): 15–e6.

Plumb, D.C. (2011). *Plumb's Veterinary Drug Handbook*, 7e. Ames, IA: Wiley Blackwell.

Reedy, L.M., Miller, W.H., and Willemese, T. (1997). *Allergic Skin Diseases of Dogs and Cats*, 2e. Philadelphia: W.B. Saunders.

Stallergenes Greer (2018). An effective way to treat allergies. http://www.greerlabs.com/index.php/veterinary_allergy/veterinary_dermatologist/ (accessed May 2015).

Zoetis (n.d.) Cytopoint®. Canine atopic dermatitis immunotherapeutic. https://www.zoetisus.com/products/dogs/cytopoint/assets/resources/cytopoint-approved-package-insert.pdf (accessed May 2019).

Zoetis (2016). Consumer package insert for Apoquel. https://www.old.health.gov.il/units/pharmacy/trufot/alonim/Rishum_4_71188217.pdf (accessed May 2019).

8

Food Hypersensitivity
Shelley Shopsowitz

Introduction

Many different terms are used when discussing what is commonly thought of as food allergy. True food allergy is an immune-mediated, reproducible, adverse response to a food antigen. Food intolerance refers to any abnormal physiological response to a food, including chocolate or onion toxicosis, reaction to vasoactive amines in some fish, and reactions to bacterial contamination of food. Since true food allergy and some food intolerances are clinically indistinguishable, the more general term adverse food reaction (AFR) is often used.

The true incidence of food allergy in the canine population is not known. Estimates range from 1 to 7% and food allergy has been proposed to cause 5–20% of all canine allergic skin disease (Carlotti 2014). Food allergy can be seen together with canine atopic dermatitis and flea allergy dermatitis and can mimic clinical signs of these other allergic diseases. One large study found that 12% of cats presented to veterinary dermatologists were diagnosed with food hypersensitivity (Hobi et al. 2011).

Food items that have been reported to cause AFRs in dogs include beef, soy, chicken, milk, corn, wheat, eggs, and fish (Miller et al. 2013). In cats, beef, dairy products, fish, lamb baby food, and clam juice have been reported (Miller et al. 2013). The ingredients most commonly found to cause AFRs generally correspond to the ingredients commonly found in commercial pet foods.

Pathogenesis

Food allergy results from a breakdown in the normal development of immunological tolerance to food antigens. Anything that increases the permeability of the gastrointestinal mucosa, for example infancy, old age, or disease, can increase the chances of sensitization to food allergens. We know little about the process in dogs and cats and most of our information is extrapolated from studies in humans. The majority of food allergy in humans is an immunoglobulin E (IgE)-mediated type I hypersensitivity response (Jackson 2014). Cell-mediated (type IV hypersensitivity) and mixed reactions have also been documented (Jackson 2014). Food allergen-specific IgE has been identified in dogs with AFRs and preliminary evidence identifying cell-mediated reactions also has been reported (Jackson 2014). The majority of food allergens in humans are glycoproteins. A heritable basis for food allergy has not been established.

Small Animal Dermatology for Technicians and Nurses, First Edition. Edited by Kim Horne, Marcia Schwassmann and Dawn Logas.
© 2020 John Wiley & Sons, Inc. Published 2020 by John Wiley & Sons, Inc.

Clinical Features

Canine AFRs can occur at any age, although many cases will be seen in dogs less than one year or older than seven years of age (Miller et al. 2013). No consistent breed predilections have been reported and males and females are affected equally.

Generalized non-seasonal pruritus is the most common sign of AFR in the dog and response to glucocorticoids is variable (Figure 8.1). Pruritus without any lesions can be seen early in the disease, but most dogs present with at least erythema or a papular dermatitis. Secondary infections with bacteria and yeast are common (Figure 8.2). Chronic cases often present with pustules, epidermal collarettes, crusting, alopecia, lichenification, and hyperpigmentation (Figure 8.3). Otitis externa usually accompanies other dermatological signs, but a small percentage of patients will present with otitis as their only sign (Figure 8.4). Any area of the body can be affected and the pattern of lesions can mimic canine atopic dermatitis

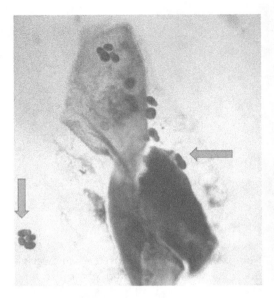

Figure 8.2 Microscopic view (100×) of a cytology sample taken from a dog with a secondary skin infection showing *malassezia* organisms (orange arrows).

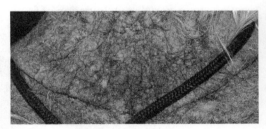

Figure 8.3 Dog diagnosed with food hypersensitivity showing chronic skin changes of hyperpigmentation and lichenification.

or, rarely, flea allergy dermatitis. There are anecdotal reports of AFRs causing recurrent superficial pyoderma without pruritus. Other less common presentations of AFRs include urticaria, angioedema, and pyotraumatic dermatitis. Some dogs with cutaneous AFRs will have concurrent gastrointestinal signs, including vomiting, diarrhea, signs of colitis, and increased frequency of bowel movements.

Cats can develop AFRs at any age, but clinical signs may start more often in younger animals (Hobi et al. 2011). There is no

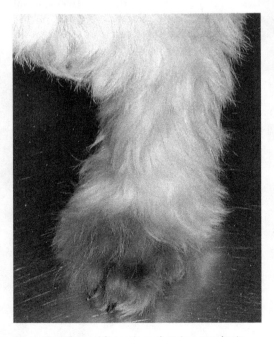

Figure 8.1 Dog with pruritus, showing porphyrin staining from licking paw.

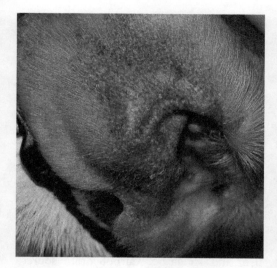

Figure 8.4 Dog with otitis externa showing pinnal erythema.

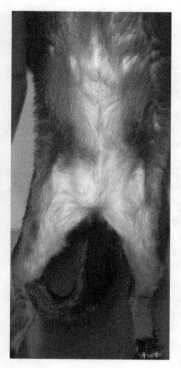

Figure 8.5 Non-inflammatory symmetric alopecia on the ventrum of a cat.

confirmed breed or sex predilection for AFRs (Hobi et al. 2011). Non-seasonal pruritus that can be severe is the most common clinical sign of AFRs. The head, face, and neck may be affected more often than in cats with environmental allergies, although this cannot be used as the sole diagnostic criterion (Hobi et al. 2011). Cats with AFRs cannot be distinguished from cats with environmental allergies or flea allergy dermatitis based on clinical signs alone. Skin lesions vary greatly and can include non-inflammatory symmetric alopecia, erythema, crusted papules, erosions/ulcerations, crusts, and eosinophilic granuloma complex lesions (lip ulcers, eosinophilic plaques, and eosinophilic granulomas) (Figures 8.5 and 8.6). Secondary bacterial and yeast infections and otitis externa may also be seen, although they are less common than in the dog. A small percentage of cats with cutaneous AFRs will also show gastrointestinal signs such as vomiting and diarrhea.

Diagnostic Tests

As with most dermatological diseases, important clues to the diagnosis can be found in the history (see Chapter 1). Clients should

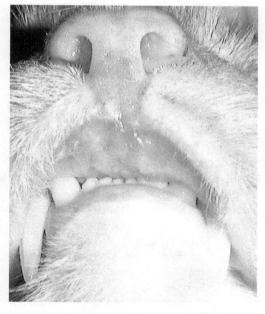

Figure 8.6 Cat presenting with eosinophilic granuloma complex lesion (indolent ulcer).

be asked how old the pet was when clinical signs started, since AFRs can start in very young or very old patients. The presence and degree of pruritus should be assessed as well as if there is any seasonality. AFRs should present with non-seasonal year-round pruritus, unless the offending food item is fed intermittently. Pets with year-round pruritus can have either AFR or atopic dermatitis or a combination of the two. Documenting pruritus in cats can be challenging, since some cats only over-groom in private. Trichograms demonstrating hairs with blunted tips can help confirm self-induced alopecia. Flea control measures should be noted, since AFRs can sometimes mimic the clinical signs of flea allergy dermatitis.

It is particularly important to obtain a complete dietary history for these patients. A list of all foods the pet has eaten as far back as the client can remember should be compiled. This includes all treats, rawhides, human food, flavored supplements, dental hygiene products, and so on that the patient consumes. Clients should be asked specifically if the pet has any gastrointestinal signs such as vomiting, diarrhea, or frequent bowel movements. Clients are often under the misconception that signs of AFRs begin soon after a diet change. They must be informed that AFRs can occur without any dietary change and that this situation is actually more common. If the patient has been placed on an elimination diet previously, it must be determined whether the diet trial was done appropriately and whether the patient improved.

The differential diagnosis list for AFRs includes parasitic disorders and other allergic diseases. The clinician will determine the appropriate diagnostic tests to rule out those conditions. Secondary bacterial and yeast infections must be identified and treated.

A definitive diagnosis of AFR can only be made via an elimination diet trial followed by dietary challenge. Both intradermal testing with food extracts and *in vitro* measurement of allergen-specific IgE and IgG levels are not accurate for the diagnosis of food allergy and should not be used.

Choosing an Elimination Diet

Diet trials can be done with novel protein diets or with hydrolyzed protein diets. Novel protein diets contain protein and carbohydrate sources to which the patient has not previously been exposed. There are a number of commercially available novel protein and carbohydrate diets that can be used for this purpose. Those diets available by prescription only are preferred due to possible contamination of over-the-counter limited-ingredient diets with proteins not listed on the ingredient labels (Raditic et al. 2011). Protein sources commonly found in these diets include venison, rabbit, duck, white fish, and kangaroo. Carbohydrate sources include potato, sweet potato, oats, and squash.

A homemade elimination diet is ideal, since home cooking can completely eliminate the risk of cross-contamination present in commercially prepared foods. A veterinary nutritionist (www.acvn.org) should be consulted to ensure the homemade diet is nutritionally complete. Unfortunately, the difficulty of obtaining the novel protein source as well as the time required to prepare a homemade diet limits the number of clients willing to use this option.

Hydrolyzed protein diets are another option for an elimination diet. These diets contain proteins that have been broken down (hydrolyzed) into smaller fragments (peptides) that are smaller than what the immune system can recognize. Hydrolyzed diet protein sources include soy, chicken, and chicken feathers. Theoretically, even a patient reactive to the intact protein should tolerate the hydrolyzed form of the protein; however, a few individuals may still react to these diets (Bizikova and Olivry 2016). There are currently a wide variety of novel protein diets available over the counter and some pets will have been exposed to many of these proteins already. Hydrolyzed diets may be a good option for these pets. Patients younger than one year of age should be fed one of the commercially prepared elimination diets labeled for growth, or a homemade diet that has been formulated by a veterinary nutritionist.

Performing the Diet Trial

The elimination diet should be fed exclusively for the duration of the trial; no other foods, treats, rawhides, table scraps, flavored toothpastes, or dietary supplements should be allowed. Chewable medications, including heartworm and flea preventatives, should be changed to non-flavored or topical products. The recommended duration of an elimination diet trial is generally two to three months. Most patients will begin to show improvement by 6 weeks, although complete resolution of signs can take up to 12 weeks (Miller et al. 2013). Treatment of secondary bacterial and yeast infections is begun simultaneously with the diet trial and is stopped once the patient's infections have cleared. Severely pruritic patients may need additional medications to relieve their discomfort. This symptomatic therapy is later withdrawn in order to evaluate the patient's response to the diet. If no improvement is seen by the end of the elimination diet trial, AFR is unlikely to be the diagnosis and other causes for the patient's pruritus should be investigated (Miller et al. 2013).

Dietary Challenge

If the patient improves on the elimination diet, they then are challenged with their previous diet to confirm the diagnosis of AFR. Clinical signs can recur as soon as 1–2 days and usually return within 7–10 days (Miller et al. 2013). If the patient does not flare upon challenge with the previous diet, AFR is not present and other reasons for improvement should be considered, for instance change of season in an atopic dog or anti-inflammatory doses of fish oil present in some elimination diets. If the patient flares, they are put back on the elimination diet to control their signs. Clients are then encouraged to complete an individual ingredient provocation trial to determine which ingredient or ingredients in

the food are the actual cause of the patient's AFR. This involves adding individual items to the elimination diet, usually one item every two weeks. Meat sources the patient has eaten previously are normally added first. Flavored heartworm and flea medications are typically included early in the challenge process. Knowing which individual ingredients the patient should avoid provides important information for clients when selecting maintenance diets for their pets.

Treatment

Once the diagnosis is confirmed, treatment of AFRs consists of feeding a diet that does not contain the offending ingredient or ingredients. Most patients can be maintained on a commercially prepared food, but a very small number of patients will only tolerate homemade diets. It is particularly important that these diets be monitored by a veterinary nutritionist to prevent nutrient, vitamin, and mineral deficiencies in these patients. Development of new food sensitivities is uncommon, but should be considered if a patient begins to flare up on a diet that they previously tolerated.

Client Education

Client participation is crucial to the diagnosis and treatment of AFRs in dogs and cats. Misconceptions and myths about "food allergies" abound and clients must receive accurate information from the veterinary staff. Some common misconceptions include that grains and gluten are a common cause of AFRs in dogs and cats, that dogs and cats cannot have allergies to diets labeled organic, that diets contain only the protein listed in the name of the food, that dogs and cats only show signs of food allergies after a diet change, that changing to a different brand of commercial dog food is an appropriate elimination diet trial, and that over-the-counter limited-ingredient diets are adequate as elimination diets. Prescription diets used for elimination diet trials are expensive and clients should be encouraged to think of these diets as a diagnostic test, not necessarily as a permanent diet change.

Once the veterinarian has chosen the diet, the veterinary technician plays an important role to ensure the diet trial is performed correctly. An elimination diet trial is a test that is performed completely by the client outside of the veterinary facility. As such, it is essential that the owner fully understands how to perform the diet trial. Written instructions (Box 8.1) that can be reviewed with the technician in the office and then taken home by the client are essential. A thorough dietary history will allow for the selection of an appropriate elimination diet.

After the diet is chosen, clients should introduce the new diet slowly to avoid gastrointestinal upset. Most of the novel protein commercial diets come in dry and canned forms. Picky eaters can be encouraged to try the new food by adding some canned food to the dry diet. Alternatively, a small amount of the selected protein can be cooked and added to increase palatability. Several different diets may need to be tried; most manufacturers guarantee their diets and have a liberal return policy.

Cats are often more challenging than dogs when trying to change diets and cats should be monitored closely to avoid hepatic lipidosis due to anorexia. Clients with multiple-cat households may need to use several different elimination diets simultaneously to ensure that all cats are eating well. Even multiple-pet households with dogs only can be challenging. It may be easier to feed all dogs the new diet, but if that is not appropriate, pets may need to be separated at feeding time and all bowls picked up afterwards. Be sure all bowls are thoroughly washed after each feeding and if clients store food in a container other than the original bag, it is preferred that they use a new container for the elimination diet. Dogs on a diet trial must not have access to cats' food or litter boxes during this period.

Strict adherence to the diet must be emphasized. Many clients mistakenly think feeding a small treat a few times a week is acceptable and it must be made clear that this is not the case. If clients are accustomed to feeding pets from the table or giving treats throughout the day, they should be encouraged to use the new food as treats. If other items are needed as treats, cooked pieces of the plain protein or carbohydrate in the diet can be used or certain treats made from the same ingredients can be used. If pets visit the groomer, day care, or other households, all people must be informed of the elimination diet trial and provided with the correct diet and treats. Free-roaming dogs and cats should be confined if at all possible to ensure compliance with dietary restrictions. Clients with young children or seniors with dementia in the house may not be able to successfully perform a strict elimination diet trial for their pet.

A list of all medications and supplements the pet takes should be reviewed and any flavored/chewable products should be replaced with non-flavored versions when possible. A small amount of the canned food or a piece of the cooked protein or carbohydrate (e.g. potato) can be used to hide pills if needed. Dogs who need something to chew on can be given Kong toys with the canned food smeared on the inside and then frozen.

Adhering to the strict diet for the full 6–12 weeks is difficult. Frequent communication with clients during this period can improve compliance. A phone call one week after the diet trial has started can help identify and correct problems early and follow-up phone calls throughout the diet trial period are recommended. Patients with secondary infections will often need rechecks before the diet trial is finished, and this is a good opportunity to assess compliance and offer encouragement.

If the patient improves on the elimination diet trial, then they need to be challenged with their previous diet to confirm the diagnosis of AFR. Treats that were fed regularly before the diet trial should also be

Box 8.1 Example of a Client Handout that can be used for Patients Starting an Elimination Diet Trial

Elimination Diet Trial Instructions

The diagnosis of food allergy is made by feeding a diet made with ingredients that your pet has never eaten before or a hydrolyzed diet (a food in which the protein is broken down into pieces too small for the immune system to recognize and react to). Switching brands of commercial dog or cat food will not accomplish this task, since many diets share common ingredients. We will recommend a specific commercial or homemade diet for your pet.

WHILE ON THE FOOD TRIAL, YOUR PET MAY NOT RECEIVE ANYTHING ELSE BY MOUTH UNLESS PRESCRIBED BY US

This means **NO** treats, rawhide chews, table scraps, chewable/flavored vitamins or other supplements, flavored toothpaste, or chewable medications (heartworm preventatives can be changed to a non-flavored or topical preventative during the course of the trial).

IT IS VERY IMPORTANT TO BE 100% STRICT DURING THE FOOD TRIAL

- Make sure all family members and friends know that your pet is on a special diet.
- If you need to use treats for rewards or training purposes, use some of the new diet or the other treats prescribed by us.
- If pills are prescribed for your pet, hide them in a small piece of the canned version of the prescribed diet. If your pet will not take the pills in this way, please contact our office for advice.
- Other pets in the household will need to be fed separately from the pet on the food trial or if the same species, be changed to the food trial diet.
- If your pet is in the habit of eating food dropped by young children, keep your pet out of the room at meal times.

- Do not let your pet lick plates or bowls and keep dogs out of cat litter boxes.

When changing over to the new food, please follow the gradual change below to avoid gastrointestinal upset. If your pet is particularly sensitive to dietary change, please let us know and we will have you do an even more gradual change to the new food.

Day 1 – ¾ of regular diet and ¼ of new diet
Day 2 – ½ of regular diet and ½ of new diet
Day 3 – ¼ of regular diet and ¾ of new diet
Day 4 – new diet only!

This diet must be fed exclusively for an 8–10-week period. Please feed the amount indicated on the packaging based on the age and body weight of your pet, unless otherwise directed by your pet's dermatologist. If your pet is gaining or losing weight, will not eat the prescribed diet, or has any problems such as vomiting or diarrhea, please contact us for advice.

Many food-allergic pets will start showing improvement in 6 weeks, but a few individuals may take 8–10 weeks to show significant improvement. Please do not give up hope and stop the food trial prematurely.

Contact our office for instructions when you see improvement or at the end of the trial. Once your pet has improved, the old diet should be re-introduced. Food allergy is confirmed if your pet flares up on his/her original diet. Individual ingredient diet challenges can also be performed. If there has not been any improvement, we will discuss the next steps.

We realize this is not an easy task, however it is our best test to diagnose or rule out a food allergy. At any time, if you have questions please contact us and we will be happy to help.

reintroduced, either together with the diet or separately. Winter is a good time to do an elimination diet trial in colder climates, as that can eliminate changing pollen levels as a confounding factor. Clients may be reluctant to challenge the diet and can be reminded that this is the only way to confirm the diagnosis. Clients should be reassured that pets can be placed back on the elimination diet as soon as they start to flare up and that they will not necessarily immediately develop clinical signs equal in severity to their previously chronic disease.

Once the diagnosis has been confirmed, clients are encouraged to do single-ingredient challenges. This provocation trial allows identification of the individual offending food items and can guide selection of a maintenance diet for the patient. A handout can be provided to the client to keep track of the challenge items and results. This process can be time consuming and labor intensive, so some clients opt to stay on the elimination diet permanently, or may try to find an over-the-counter diet with similar ingredients to use as a maintenance diet. Most pets can be maintained on the same elimination diet long term. Development of new food sensitivities is unusual, but should be considered if patients begin to have problems again. Clients should be questioned carefully to determine if the patient has received any different food items that could account for the flare-up. Symptomatic therapy may be required if breaks in strict diet adherence occur.

Conclusion

Despite the fact that little is known about the pathophysiology of AFRs in animals, the condition has an excellent prognosis assuming the offending food item or items can be consistently avoided. Occasional exposures can usually be managed with symptomatic therapy for the pruritus and treatment of secondary infections. The increase in the number of prescription diets suitable for elimination diet trials has made diagnosis of the disease easier, while the proliferation of over-the-counter diets containing unusual proteins has made selection of a novel protein for some patients more difficult. Client participation is more important for the diagnosis and management of AFRs than perhaps any other allergic skin disease. Thorough client education can ensure a good outcome for these patients.

References

Bizikova, P. and Olivry, T. (2016). A randomized, double-blinded crossover trial testing the benefits of two hydrolysed poultry-based commercial diets for dogs with spontaneous pruritic chicken allergy. *Veterinary Dermatology* 27: 289–e70.

Carlotti, D.N. (2014). Cutaneous manifestations of food hypersensitivity. In: *Veterinary Allergy* (eds. C. Noli, A. Foster and W. Rosenkrantz), 108–114. Chichester: Wiley.

Hobi, S., Linek, M., Marignac, G. et al. (2011). Clinical characteristics and causes of pruritus in cats: a multicentre study on feline hypersensitivity-associated dermatoses. *Veterinary Dermatology* 22: 406–413.

Jackson, H.A. (2014). The pathogenesis of food allergy. In: *Veterinary Allergy* (eds. C. Noli, A. Foster and W. Rosenkrantz), 103–107. Chichester: Wiley.

Miller, W.H., Griffin, C.E., and Campbell, K.L. (2013). *Muller and Kirk's Small Animal Dermatology*, 7e. St. Louis, MO: Elsevier.

Raditic, D.M., Remillard, R.L., and Tater, K.C. (2011). ELISA testing for common food antigens in four dry dog foods used in dietary elimination trials. *Journal of Animal Physiology and Animal Nutrition* 95: 90–97.

Section IV

Parasitic Skin Diseases

9

Sarcoptic Mange
Stephanie B. Duggan

Introduction

Sarcoptic mange (scabies, sarcoptic acariasis) is a contagious, non-seasonal, intensely pruritic dermatitis caused by infestation with the mite *Sarcoptes scabiei*. These mites can be difficult to find on skin scrapings, since there may only be small numbers of mites on an affected individual. This makes it easy to miss the diagnosis, especially since the clinical signs of sarcoptic mange can look similar to food allergy, atopic dermatitis, contact dermatitis, cheyletiellosis, *malassezia* dermatitis, and other inflammatory skin diseases.

A treatment trial should be performed to rule out this disease when a patient has compatible clinical signs, even if skin scrapings are negative. Failing to do so can lead to unnecessary suffering for the patient and frustration for the owner. Sarcoptic mange should be considered more likely when a patient's onset of pruritus is acute, if the pruritus is severe and continuous, if the pruritus does not respond to conventional therapies, and if other animals/people in the home are affected.

Pathogenesis

S. scabiei var. *canis* is found most commonly on domestic dogs and wild canids such as foxes and coyotes. Each variant of *S. scabiei* has host preferences, but can infect a variety of mammalian species. Therefore all canids in contact with the affected dog should be treated and owners should be warned of the zoonotic nature of the disease. Canine scabies is usually a self-limiting disease in humans; however, any owners affected should be referred to their physician for advice.

Feline scabies is caused by *Notoedres cati*, a different sarcoptiform mite. The disease is also highly contagious and pruritic, but in contrast to canine scabies, these mites are usually present in large numbers so are easily found on skin scrapings.

Adult *S. scabiei* var. *canis* mites are round to oval shaped, 200–400 μm in length, with four pairs of short legs, and a terminally located anus. The front two pairs of legs have long, unjointed stalks with terminal suckers (Figure 9.1). Adult *N. cati* mites are slightly smaller, have medium-length stalks with terminal suckers, and have a dorsally located anus (Figure 9.2). The life cycles of both mites are thought to be similar. The adult females tunnel through the superficial layers of the epidermis and lay eggs in the tunnels. The eggs proceed through one larval and two nymphal stages before molting into adults. The entire life cycle can be completed in 14–21 days, depending on environmental conditions. The mites usually spend their entire life on the host, but they can survive in the environment for a short period of time.

Small Animal Dermatology for Technicians and Nurses, First Edition. Edited by Kim Horne, Marcia Schwassmann and Dawn Logas.

(a)

(b)

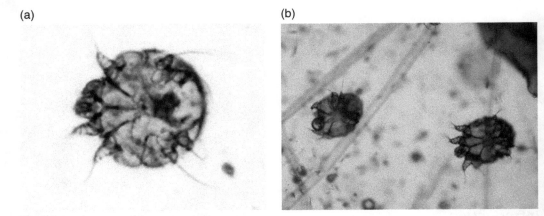

Figures 9.1 (a and b) Skin scrapings showing adult *Sarcoptes scabiei* mites with non-segmented legs with a sucker on the end.

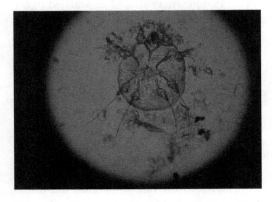

Figure 9.2 Skin scraping showing an adult notoedric mite. *Source:* Photo by Dr. Clarissa Souza, courtesy of Universidade Federal Rural do Rio de Janeiro, Brazil.

Under ideal temperature and humidity conditions, *S. scabiei* var. *canis* females and nymphs can survive in the environment for a few weeks, therefore thorough cleaning is recommended and treatment of the environment with parasiticidal sprays may be indicated (Miller et al. 2013).

The mite is believed to cause a hypersensitivity reaction in the host that is responsible for the severe pruritus. The exact incubation period is not known, but onset of signs usually occurs within days of exposure (Miller et al. 2013). The disease is highly contagious and indirect transmission via grooming equipment, bedding, and fur can occur.

Clinical Features

The classic canine scabies patient presents with a sudden onset of an intensely pruritic, papular, crusting dermatitis affecting the face, ear pinnae, elbows, hocks, and ventrum (Figures 9.3 and 9.4). If left untreated, chronic inflammation and self-trauma can lead to the development of excoriations, thick yellow crusting, alopecia, lichenification, and hyper-pigmentation (Figures 9.5 and 9.6). Lesions can become generalized and severely affected dogs can show weight loss and generalized lymphadenopathy. Secondary bacterial infections are common and may necessitate antibiotic therapy in addition to miticidal therapy.

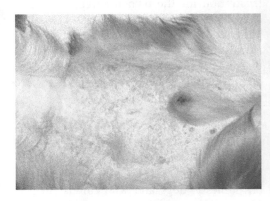

Figure 9.3 Dog with sarcoptic mange showing clinical signs of papules and alopecia on ventral abdomen.

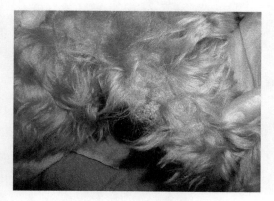

Figure 9.4 Dog with sarcoptic mange showing clinical signs of crusting and erythema on elbow.

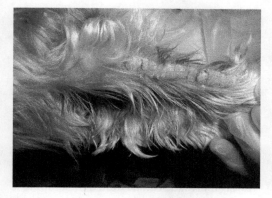

Figure 9.5 Dog with sarcoptic mange showing clinical signs of crusting, alopecia, erythema, and lichenification on ear pinna.

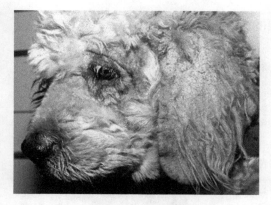

Figure 9.6 Dog with sarcoptic mange showing clinical signs of crusting, scaling, lichenification, and alopecia.

Sarcoptic mange is most often seen in younger dogs, but no breed or sex predilections have been documented; therefore a good patient history becomes even more important to obtaining the diagnosis. A history of contact with an infected animal is helpful, but suspicion should also increase if the patient has more opportunity for contact with other animals by being boarded, visiting dog parks, hunting, attending dog shows, or going to the groomer. Contact with wildlife, especially wild canids, as well as the presence of other affected pets or humans in the household, should also increase suspicion of sarcoptic mange. However, lack of an obvious source of the mite infestation should not by itself rule out the possibility of sarcoptic mange as a diagnosis. It is not unusual for patients diagnosed with sarcoptic mange to have no known history of exposure.

Some patients with scabies show minimal to no response to glucocorticoid therapy, so it is important to ask owners what the pet has been treated with previously and what was the pet's response to therapy.

Feline scabies (notoedric mange) is an intensely pruritic, papular dermatitis typically affecting the ear pinnae, face, neck, feet, and perineum (Miller et al. 2013). Severe crusting develops rapidly and with chronicity, lichenification, excoriations, and alopecia can become generalized (Figures 9.7 and 9.8). Like its canine counterpart, it is highly contagious and has no age, breed, or sex predilections.

Diagnostic Tests

The diagnosis of sarcoptic mange is confirmed by finding any mites, eggs, or fecal pellets on superficial skin scrapings (Figures 9.9 and 9.10). The veterinary technician should be familiar with the appearance of sarcoptes eggs and fecal pellets, as they are diagnostic if found on the scraping, even if no mites are seen. Scabies mites can be difficult to find, so multiple, broad, superficial

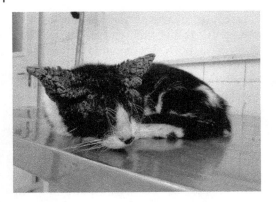

Figure 9.7 Cat with notoedric mange showing severe crusting on pinnae. *Source:* Photo by Dr. Clarissa Souza, courtesy of Universidade Federal Rural do Rio de Janeiro, Brazil.

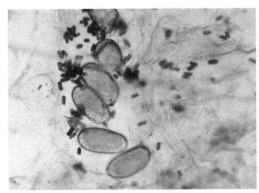

Figure 9.10 Skin scraping showing *Sarcoptes scabiei* eggs and fecal pellets.

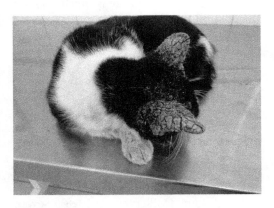

Figure 9.8 Cat with notoedric mange showing severe crusting on pinnae. *Source:* Photo by Dr. Clarissa Souza, courtesy of Universidade Federal Rural do Rio de Janeiro, Brazil.

skin scrapings should be performed and negative skin scrapings do not rule out the diagnosis. Clinically affected areas should be scraped. Papular, crusted areas on the ear pinnae, elbows, and hocks are good locations to scrape. Heavily excoriated areas should be avoided, as they typically do not yield mites.

Multiple superficial scrapings should be performed on the affected areas with a spatula (Figure 9.11) or dull #10 scalpel blade. The scalpel blade can be dulled by scraping it on the side of a metal exam table. A small amount of mineral oil is placed on the spatula or scalpel blade and may also be applied to the sites to be scraped. Coating the spatula or

(a)

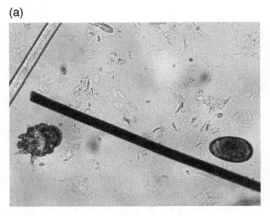

(b)

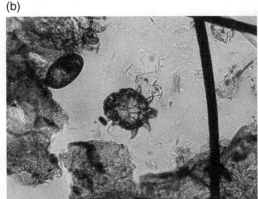

Figure 9.9 (a and b) Skin scrapings showing an adult *Sarcoptes scabiei* mite and egg.

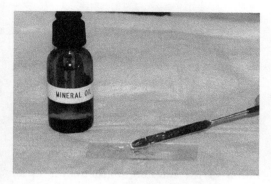

Figure 9.11 Spatula, mineral oil, and slide used for skin scrapings.

blade with mineral oil allows the collected debris to adhere to the scraping instrument. Select sites and scrape over a broad area. Scabies mites live in the superficial layers of the epidermis, so deep scrapings are not needed to find the mites. Place the collected scale and debris on the slide, then place a cover slip on top of the material. More mineral oil may need to be applied to the slide to allow adequate spreading of the sample. Too thick a layer of debris can make visualization of mites more difficult. All areas of the slide should be carefully examined under low power (4× or 10× objective), with the condenser lowered to increase contrast. Feline scabies (notoedric mange) is much easier to diagnose, as the mites are usually present in large numbers and are easily found on skin scraping.

Scabies mites are occasionally observed in fecal flotations when the host ingests mites during the intensive licking and chewing caused by the disease; therefore, a fecal exam may be another diagnostic option. Serologic testing by enzyme-linked immunosorbent assay (ELISA) for immunoglobulin G (IgG) antibodies to sarcoptes mites is available in Europe and can be a useful diagnostic aid (Foster and Foil 2003; Miller et al. 2013). Histopathological findings are usually non-specific and only in very rare cases are mites seen in biopsy specimens from canine scabies (Medleau and Hnilica 2001).

A positive pinnal–pedal reflex supports the diagnosis of scabies, but is not specific for the disease. This test is positive if the hind leg reaches to scratch at the ear when the edge of the ear pinna is rubbed or scratched.

If the diagnosis cannot be confirmed by the methods listed above, a therapeutic trial should be performed. A negative response to scabicidal therapy is the only way to exclude scabies from the differential diagnosis list.

Treatment

Some infected dogs will develop an immune response to the mites that may eventually result in spontaneous resolution of the disease (Foster and Foil 2003; Miller et al. 2013). However, treatment is still recommended due to the contagious and pruritic nature of sarcoptic mange.

There are many different treatment options available for sarcoptic mange. Client and patient factors will help determine which therapy is best for each individual. In addition to scabicidal agents, some clinicians will also prescribe a short course of glucocorticoids to decrease the intense pruritus that may persist for multiple days. Systemic antibiotics may be prescribed if secondary bacterial infection is present, and an antiseborrheic or antibacterial shampoo may be recommended to remove crusts and treat secondary infections.

Topically active miticidal therapies include 2–4% lime sulfur dips (approved in North America) and 0.025% amitraz dips (approved in the United Kingdom). Lime sulfur dips are applied once a week for four to six weeks (Foster and Foil 2003; Miller et al. 2013). Long coats should be clipped short to facilitate contact of the dipping solution with the skin and the entire body surface of the patient must be treated. Lime sulfur is an extremely safe therapy; however, the dip smells of sulfur, temporarily stains light-colored haircoats yellow, and discolors jewelry and porcelain. Label precautions for owners and patients must be carefully followed when using amitraz dips and the drug is not approved for use in cats, pregnant dogs, and puppies under four months of age (Pharmacia and Upjohn 2007).

Fipronil (Frontline Spray®, Merial Animal Health, Lyon, France) is label approved as an aid to controlling sarcoptic mange infestations in dogs. It may be best used for early, mild cases, or when other therapies are not appropriate (Curtis 2004).

Systemically active miticidal agents include ivermectin, milbemycin oxime, selamectin, moxidectin, afoxolaner, fluralaner, and sarolaner. Ivermectin can be administered orally, topically, or by subcutaneous injection. Two to three treatments at 14-day intervals or four to six treatments at 7-day intervals are generally recommended (Burrows 2009). The recommended dose range is 0.2–0.4 mg/kg. Collies and other herding breeds can have an increased sensitivity to ivermectin toxicity and scabicidal doses of ivermectin can cause depression, ataxia, mydriasis, blindness, bradycardia, muscle tremors, disorientation, coma, and death in these individuals. Their increased sensitivity is due to a mutation in the ABCB1 (formerly MDR1) gene that allows greater concentrations of ivermectin to enter the mammalian brain. Screening for this genetic mutation can be done through the Washington State University Veterinary Clinical Pathology Laboratory (www.vetmed.wsu.edu/depts-VCPL/test.aspx; Burrows 2009).

Milbemycin oxime at a dose of 2 mg/kg can be given orally at 7-day intervals for three to five treatments and is generally safe for use in ivermectin-sensitive breeds. Some collies are sensitive to higher doses of milbemycin, so accurate dosing is important.

Selamectin (Revolution®, Zoetis, Parsippany, NJ) is available in a topical spot-on formulation licensed for the treatment and control of sarcoptic mange in dogs when used at the labeled dose of 6–12 mg/kg once every 30 days. Many dermatologists recommend three treatments at two-week intervals for increased therapeutic efficacy. This dose of selamectin has been shown to be safe in avermectin-sensitive collies.

Moxidectin is available as a 2.5% topical spot-on formulation (in combination with imidacloprid) labeled for the treatment and control of sarcoptic mange in dogs. Once-a-month application is the label-approved dose, but, as with selamectin, many dermatologists will recommend three treatments at two-week intervals to ensure complete resolution of the infestation (McKeever et al. 2009). Moxidectin in this form is safe for use in ivermectin-sensitive collies as long as it is not ingested. The large animal injectable formulation of moxidectin can be given orally or by subcutaneous injection at 0.2–0.25 mg/kg once a week for three to six treatments for the treatment of sarcoptic mange (Burrows 2009). This dosage is not safe for use in ivermectin-sensitive breeds.

Afoxalaner (NexGard®, Boehringer Ingelheim, Duluth, GA), fluralaner (Bravecto®, Merck Animal Health, Madison, NJ), and sarolaner (Simparica®, Zoetis) are all members of a newer class of parasiticides called isoxazolines. They are all labeled for control of fleas and ticks, but have also shown good efficacy for treatment of scabies infestations in dogs (Becskei et al. 2016; Beugnet et al. 2016; Romero et al. 2016; Taenzler et al. 2016). Afoxalaner and sarolaner are administered orally once a month. Fluralaner is administered once every three months and is available in both oral and topical formulations for dogs.

Treatment of feline scabies (notoedric mange) is similar to the treatment of canine scabies. Once-weekly 2–3% lime sulfur dips, selamectin (three treatments at two-week intervals), ivermectin (0.2–0.4 mg/kg orally or by subcutaneous injection every one to two weeks for four to six weeks), and doramectin have all been recommended for treatment (Burrows 2009; Kennis 2004). Other than lime sulfur dips, all the treatments mentioned constitute off-label use of the drugs. Fluralaner (Bravecto) has recently been released as a topical flea control product for cats. At the time of writing of this chapter, no published data regarding the effectiveness of fluralaner for the treatment of feline scabies was available.

Because scabies mites can survive in the environment for up to three weeks, environmental cleaning and scabicidal treatment may be recommended in multiple-pet households or if numerous mites are found on a pet. Weekly washing of the pet's bedding and grooming equipment, as well as regular vacuuming and mopping of floors, are recommended. The clinician may also recommend treating the environment with parasiticidal sprays.

Care must also be taken to avoid spreading scabies in the veterinary hospital. Protective clothing should be worn when handling patients with suspected scabies and good hand washing should always take place before and after handling patients. Patients with confirmed or suspected sarcoptic mange should be isolated and the areas they occupied should be thoroughly cleaned and treated with parasiticidal agents as necessary.

Client Education

The contagious and zoonotic nature of sarcoptic mange must be emphasized to clients. They must understand that all in-contact dogs need to be treated simultaneously and that environmental treatment may also be required. Owners should be instructed to keep affected animals isolated to avoid spreading the disease. Visits to boarding facilities, doggie day care, play groups, dog parks, and the groomer should be postponed until treatment is completed. Clients should also be advised to contact their physician if they have lesions.

Proper administration of each treatment method must be explained to owners. If dips are being used, consider clipping pets with long and thick coats to ensure contact of the dip with the skin. Bathing prior to dipping is often recommended to remove thick crust and scale from the skin surface prior to applying the miticidal agent. Some patients may need to wear an Elizabethan collar until they are dry to prevent them from licking off and ingesting the dip. Make sure the owners know that the dip must be applied to the entire animal, including the head, ears, and face, taking care to avoid getting dip into the eyes. Some owners will prefer the treatment be performed by the veterinary hospital and this should be encouraged, as proper application of the dip can be ensured. The number of treatments needed must be made clear and clients must finish the series of dips, even if their pet is considerably improved before treatment is completed.

Proper application of spot-on formulations should be explained to the owner. The product must be applied to the skin, not on top of the haircoat, and animals should not be allowed to lick the area where the product is applied. Animals should not be bathed, usually for several days after the product has been applied. Consult each product's label for specific recommendations. How often to apply the product and for how long must be made clear, especially if the directions for scabicidal use differ from the product label. Remember to also advise clients if the spot-on being used has other applications such as flea and heartworm prevention. Some of the spot-on formulations may require a negative heartworm test before their use can be recommended. Proper administration of oral medications, especially liquids, should be explained to ensure the patient receives the entire dose of the medication. Informed consent must be obtained from owners whenever off-label use of medications is being recommended. The veterinarian and veterinary staff must make sure owners are aware of the potential adverse effects of each treatment and what to do if adverse effects are noted.

Some dermatologists report an initial temporary increase in pruritus after treatment is started. A hypersensitivity reaction to dying mites has been proposed as the reason for this pruritus, but this theory remains unproven. Owners should be informed of this possibility to avoid premature discontinuation of treatment.

Conclusion

Unlike many of the diseases seen by dermatologists, sarcoptic mange is a curable disease. However, because the mite can be hard to find, this condition is often undiagnosed or misdiagnosed as allergies. Performing a treatment trial in any patient with suggestive history and clinical signs is a good first step. If there is no response to the treatment trial, then further work-up to diagnose the patient's problem should be pursued.

Many effective miticidal therapies are available today. The veterinary technician, through detailed and complete client education, can ensure that the treatment plan is followed and successful resolution of the disease is achieved.

References

Becskei, C., DeBock, F., Illambas, J. et al. (2016). Efficacy and safety of a novel isoxazoline, sarolaner (Simparica™), for the treatment of sarcoptic mange in dogs. *Veterinary Parasitology* 222: 56–61.

Beugnet, F., de Vos, C., Liebenberg, J. et al. (2016). Efficacy of afoxolaner in a clinincal field study in dogs naturally infested with *Sarcoptes scabiei. Parasite* 23: 26.

Burrows, A. (2009). Avermectins in dermatology. In: *Kirk's Current Veterinary Therapy XIV* (eds. J.D. Bonagura and D.C. Twedt), 390–394. Philadelphia, PA: Saunders.

Curtis, C.F. (2004). Current trends in the treatment of Sarcoptes, Cheyletiella, otodectes mite infestation in dogs and cats. *Veterinary Dermatology* 15 (2): 108–114.

Foster, A.P. and Foil Carol, S. (2003). *BSAVA Manual of Small Animal Dermatology*, 3e. Gloucester: British Small Animal Veterinary Association.

Kennis, R. (2004). Parasiticides in dermatology. In: *Small Animal Dermatology Secrets* (ed. K. Campbell), 65. Philadeplhia: Hanley and Belfus.

McKeever, P., Nuttall, T., and Harvey, R. (2009). Pruritic dermatoses. In: *Skin Diseases of the Dog and Cat*, 2e (eds. N.A. Heinrich, M. Eisenschenk, R.G. Harvey and T. Nuttall). London: Manson Publishing, Chapter 2.

Medleau, L. and Hnilica, K. (eds.) (2001). Parasitic skin diseases. In: *Small Animal Dermatology*. Philadelphia, PA: W.B. Saunders Company, Chapter 5.

Miller, W.H., Griffin, C.E., and Campbell, K.L. (eds.) (2013). Parasitic skin diseases. In: *Muller and Kirk's Small Animal Dermatology*, 7e. St. Louis, MO: Elsevier/Mosby, Chapter 4.

Pharmacia and Upjohn, Bayley, A.J. (ed.) (2007). Mitaban product insert. In: *Compendium of Veterinary Products*, 10e. Port Huron, MI: North American Compendium.

Romero, C., Heredia, R., Pineda, J. et al. (2016). Efficacy of fluralaner in 17 dogs with sarcoptic mange. *Veterinary Dermatology* 27: 353–e88.

Taenzler, J., Liebenberg, J., Roepke, R.K.A. et al. (2016). Efficacy of fluralaner administered either orally or topically for the treatment of naturally acquired *Sarcoptes scabiei* var. *canis* infestation in dogs. *Parasites & Vectors* 9: 392.

10

Cheyletiellosis

Jennie Tait

Introduction

Cheyletiellosis (also known as *Cheyletiella* dermatitis) is a highly contagious, parasitic dermatosis caused by mites of the genus *Cheyletiella*. The disease is uncommon, but its true incidence may be underestimated since the mites can be difficult to find, are susceptible to most flea adulticides, and asymptomatic carriers are reported.

Pathogenesis

Cheyletiella mites affect a variety of species, including cats, dogs, and rabbits. These highly contagious mites are seen more often in young animals, animals in shelters, cats in catteries, and animals who visit grooming establishments and dog parks. *Cheyletiella* mites can also transiently infest people, causing a pruritic, papular dermatitis (Figure 10.1). The disease is less common in warmer climates where year-round flea control is practiced.

Cheyletiella spp. are large (500 × 350 μm) mites with four pairs of legs with terminal combs. Their most distinguishing feature is the pair of prominent hooks on the accessory mouthparts (Figure 10.2). These surface-dwelling mites feed on tissue fluid and lymph obtained by piercing the skin surface. While *Cheyletiella yasguri* is most often associated with dogs, *Cheyletiella blakei* with cats, and

Cheyletiella parasitovorax with rabbits, the mites are not completely host specific and can move easily between different host species (Figures 10.3–10.5).

All life stages of the mite occur on the host (Miller et al. 2013). Females attach their eggs to hair shafts with fine threads. After hatching, the six-legged larvae go through two eight-legged nymphal stages before emerging as adults. The entire life cycle can be completed in three to four weeks (Table 10.1).

Adult female mites are able to survive off the host for at least 10 days (Miller et al. 2013) and these adults as well as eggs that are attached to shed hairs can be a source of reinfestation. Therefore, treatment of the environment may be necessary to completely eliminate the mites, especially in multiple-pet households or severe infestations. In addition, transmission of the disease via fomites such as brushes, leashes, clothing, toys, and bedding must be avoided (Curtis and Paradis 2003).

Clinical Features

Clinical signs of cheyletiellosis are variable, ranging from minimal scaling unnoticed by owners, to severe pruritus, scaling, erythema, and papules. The most common clinical features of the disease are dry scale that is most severe on the dorsum with

Small Animal Dermatology for Technicians and Nurses, First Edition. Edited by Kim Horne,
Marcia Schwassmann and Dawn Logas.
© 2020 John Wiley & Sons, Inc. Published 2020 by John Wiley & Sons, Inc.

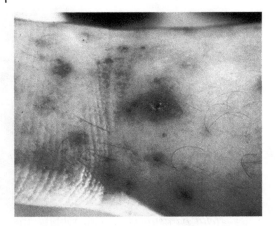

Figure 10.1 Cheyletiella dermatitis on a human arm.

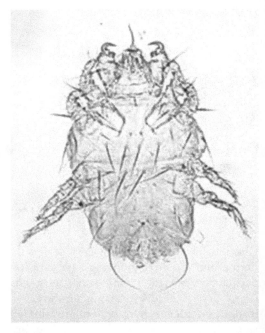

Figure 10.4 *Cheyletiella blakei* from a cat.

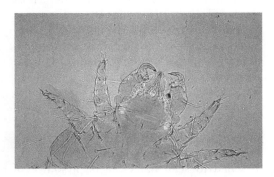

Figure 10.2 Hooked accessory mouth parts and combs on ends of legs.

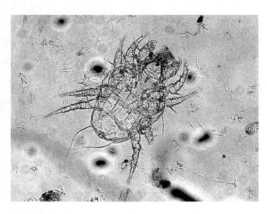

Figure 10.3 *Cheyletiella yasguri* from a dog.

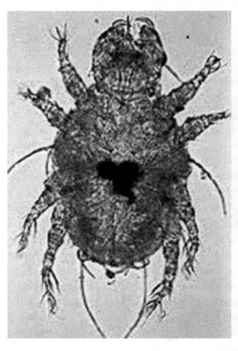

Figure 10.5 *Cheyletiella parasitovorax* from a rabbit.

Table 10.1 *Cheyletiella* life stages.

Egg	Larva	Nymph I	Nymph II	Adult
Attached by fine strands to hair shaft	6 legs	8 legs Appearance of a very small adult	8 legs Appearance of a small adult	8 legs Large adult moves rapidly
White	White	White	White to yellow	Yellowish
Hatches in 4 days	Molts in 7 days	Molts in 4½ days	Molts in 5 days	Life span of 14 days

Source: Walking dandruff, *Boxer Parade Magazine*, Summer 1979, 2(1). http://northernontarioboxerclub.com/Health.html

Figure 10.6 Close-up of scale on a dog with cheyletiella dermatitis.

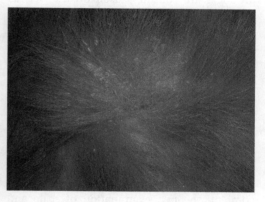

Figure 10.7 Close-up of scale on a rabbit with cheyletiella dermatitis.

mild to moderate pruritus. Patients with chronic or severe infestations may develop varying degrees of alopecia and secondary skin infections (Figure 10.6). Cats, because of their normal grooming behavior, often present with less scale than dogs. Cheyletiellosis in cats may also present as a papular, crusting eruption (miliary dermatitis), or as self-induced alopecia without any skin lesions.

Cheyletiella mites often produce no signs in rabbits. Severe infestations or sensitive individuals may show varying degrees of pruritus, scaling, crusting, alopecia, and erythema (Figure 10.7). Lesions are typically present on the dorsum and ventral abdomen (Miller et al. 2013).

Cheyletiellosis has no breed or sex predilections, but is seen more often in young animals. Debilitated animals and those housed in crowded, unsanitary conditions are also more susceptible to infestation. Pets with a history of contact with other animals, even if those animals have no signs of skin disease, are at greater risk for contracting cheyletiellosis. Because *Cheyletiella* spp. easily move between different host species, any history of contact with dogs, cats, or rabbits is significant. Owners should be asked if their pet visits grooming establishments, kennels, dog parks, dog or cat shows, or any other location where they contact other animals.

Because asymptomatic carriers exist, the disease may become apparent after introduction of a new pet into the household. The asymptomatic carrier can be the new pet or the pet already in residence. In either situation, all pets in the household must be treated to successfully eliminate the infestation. The presence of lesions on humans in the household also increases suspicion for cheyletiellosis. A person with lesions may be advised by their physician to have their pets examined by a veterinarian to determine if they are the source of the mites. Owners should be asked when the pet was last groomed or bathed, since these activities can remove mites and make diagnosis more difficult. It is also important to note which flea control products are routinely used on the pet, as some flea adulticides kill *Cheyletiella* mites while others do not.

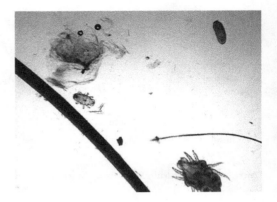

Figure 10.8 Skin scraping showing an egg, six-legged nymph, and eight-legged adult of *Cheyletiella*.

Diagnostic Tests

The diagnosis of cheyletiellosis is confirmed by identifying either mites or eggs on the pet. A variety of techniques are used to find the mites, including direct examination of the patient with a hand-held magnifying lens, examination of scale and hair collected by flea combing the pet, examination of scale and hair collected by acetate tape impression, superficial skin scrapings, and fecal flotation. Direct examination of the patient is likely to be successful only in severe infestations with large numbers of mites. Flea combing the patient allows collection of scale and hair from larger areas, increasing the chances of finding mites. The collected material can be transferred to a petri dish (with or without mineral oil) and examined with a dissecting microscope or magnifying lens, since the mites and eggs are large and easily seen. Alternatively, the hair and scale can be suspended in mineral oil on one or more slides, and then examined under low power (4x and 10x objectives) on a standard microscope. Small strips of acetate tape can be pressed repeatedly onto the skin surface to collect hair and scale. The tape is then placed on a slide with mineral oil and examined under low power (4x and 10x objectives). Multiple acetate tape preparations should be examined to increase the chances of

finding the mites. Superficial skin scrapings can also be used to collect surface scale and hair. In animals with thick, long coats, the hair should be trimmed short with scissors in the areas to be scraped to allow better access to the skin surface. Multiple scrapings of large areas will increase the chances of finding the mites (Figure 10.8). Mites or eggs may occasionally be seen on fecal flotations, especially in cats because of their self-grooming behavior. If mites are not found on the patient, consider examining other pets in the household, since asymptomatic carriers exist.

Even with intensive searching, mites may not be found in some cases. Separate studies reported failure to identify mites in 15% of dogs and 58% of cats who were infested (Paradis et al. 1990; Paradis and Villeneuve 1988). Therefore, trial miticidal therapy is indicated if clinical suspicion for the disease exists. Failure to respond to miticidal therapy is the only way to definitively rule out cheyletiellosis as a differential diagnosis.

Treatment

Although cheyletiellosis can be a challenging infestation to eliminate, particularly in multi-animal households, the disease is completely curable and has an excellent prognosis. Successful elimination of an infestation requires treatment of the patient, all in-contact pets, and in some cases the environment. Environmental treatment ranges from routine weekly house cleaning and washing pets' bedding in hot water, to spraying the house weekly with pyrethroid sprays. The degree of environmental treatment required depends on the severity of the infestation, the chronicity of the infestation, and the number of pets in the household. Grooming equipment, plush toys, pet clothing, or bedding that cannot be washed or sprayed with pyrethroid sprays should be discarded.

There are currently no veterinary products labeled for the treatment of *Cheyletiella* dermatitis; therefore, client consent should be obtained for off-label use of the treatment selected for each patient. A variety of topical and systemic drugs are effective against *Cheyletiella* mites. Patient species, breed, age, disease severity, and client preference will dictate product selection.

Weekly application of lime sulfur dips, pyrethrin dips or sprays, pyrethroid dips or sprays, or amitraz dips are all effective against *Cheyletiella* mites. Recommendations for duration of treatment range from four to eight weeks. Lime sulfur dips (3.1%) can be used on dogs, cats, and rabbits. Cats and occasionally dogs may need to wear an Elizabethan collar until they dry to prevent excessive self-grooming and ingestion of the dip. Lime sulfur is safe even for puppies and kittens, but it is drying, has an unpleasant smell, temporarily stains light-colored coats yellow, and can discolor jewelry, porcelain, and other porous surfaces (see also the handout in Box 10.1). These characteristics often make lime sulfur an unpopular choice with clients. Pyrethrin sprays and dips can be used on dogs, cats, and rabbits, but higher-concentration pyrethroids (synthetic pyrethrins) should not be used on cats and rabbits as they are more sensitive to their toxic effects. Amitraz is labeled for use in dogs only for the treatment of generalized demodicosis. It is effective against *Cheyletiella* mites, but other safer and more convenient therapies are generally recommended.

Animals with long, thick coats may need clipping before treatments begin to facilitate contact of the miticidal agent with the skin. If animals are severely affected, bathing to remove excessive crust and scale may also be advised prior to dipping. Care must be taken to ensure the dip or spray covers the entire animal or untreated areas may act as sources for continued infestation. Puppies, kittens, rabbits, and toy dog breeds must be kept warm to avoid hypothermia after dipping. The technician should discuss in detail with the owner the recommended procedure for product application. If treatments are being performed in the hospital, all staff should be made aware of the contagious nature of the pet's condition.

The 0.25% spray formulation and 10% spot-on formulation of fipronil have been shown to be effective against *Cheyletiella* mites in dogs and cats. The spray is used at one to two pumps per pound every two weeks for three to four treatments, and the spot-on formulation is applied once a month for three treatments. The spot-on formulation is sometimes used every two weeks in an attempt to achieve resolution of clinical signs more quickly (Ghubash 2006). The spray or spot-on formulation of fipronil, used every three weeks for two applications, has been recommended for cats (Guaguere 1999). Other references report the effectiveness of a single application of fipronil in the spray or spot-on formulation (Miller et al. 2013). Fipronil is toxic to rabbits and its use should be avoided in that species.

Systemically active products effective against *Cheyletiella* mites include selamectin, ivermectin, and milbemycin. Three doses of a topical spot-on formulation of selamectin applied once a month have been used successfully in cats and would be expected to work similarly in dogs (Chailleux and Paradis 2002). The injectable and oral solutions of ivermectin labeled for use in large animals are used to treat cheyletiellosis in dogs, cats, and rabbits. A dose of 0.2–0.3 mg/kg given by subcutaneous injection every two weeks for three to four treatments or orally once a week

---

Box 10.1 Client Education Handout

Cheyletiellosis

What is cheyletiellosis?

Cheyletiellosis is a skin disease of dogs, cats, and rabbits caused by *Cheyletiella* mites. These mites often cause excessive scaling/dandruff and sometimes the scale appears to be moving – hence the common name for the disease, "walking dandruff."

What is the life cycle of *Cheyletiella* mites and how are they transmitted?

The entire life cycle, from egg to adult, takes place on the host animal and can be completed in 3 weeks. *Cheyletiella* mites can be transmitted by direct contact between animals, or by contact with brushes, bedding, blankets, clothing, and plush toys. Eggs attached to hairs that have been shed into the environment can also be a source of infestation. It is therefore very important to clean and treat the environment, pet bedding, and all pets in the household at the same time, otherwise reinfestation may occur.

What are the signs of cheyletiellosis?

These mites can cause skin irritation, usually along the back of the animal. Infested animals may show mild to severe scaling/dandruff, crusting, hair loss, itching, redness, and rashes. Some animals may not show any signs of infestation.

How is an infestation with *Cheyletiella* diagnosed?

Mites may be seen on your pet, especially with the use of a magnifying glass. Examining dandruff, hairs, coat brushings, or scrapings of the skin under the microscope can positively identify the mites. Because cats groom a lot, *Cheyletiella* infestations can sometimes be diagnosed by examining their feces for the presence of *Cheyletiella* mites or eggs. Sometimes *Cheyletiella* mites can be hard to find, so your veterinarian may recommend treatment even if mites are not found on your pet.

What is the treatment for cheyletiellosis?

Cheyletiella mites are killed by many of the insecticides that are used against fleas. A treatment protocol that is most appropriate for your pet and your home environment will be recommended. Make sure we are aware of all animals in contact with your pet so they can receive the necessary treatment.

Can I get *Cheyletiella* mites from my pet?

These mites can temporarily infest humans, causing skin irritation, rashes, and itching. Treatment of your pets and the environment usually resolves the problem. Please contact your physician if you experience any symptoms that concern you.

---

for six treatments is used for dogs and cats (Burrows 2009; Ghubash 2006). Caution should be used in kittens, as they are more sensitive to the toxic effects of ivermectin (Burrows 2009). The recommended dose of ivermectin in rabbits is 0.4 mg/kg given by subcutaneous injection every 7–10 days for three treatments (Meredith 2006). These high doses of ivermectin are not safe for use in collies and other ivermectin-sensitive breeds, so alternative therapies should be chosen (see Chapters 9 and 11 for additional

information on ivermectin sensitivity testing). A topical pour-on formulation of ivermectin applied every two weeks for four treatments was also effective against cheyletiellosis in cats (Page et al. 2000). Milbemycin oxime, 2 mg/kg given orally once a week for a minimum of three weeks, was shown to be effective against *Cheyletiella* mites in dogs (Burrows 2009; Miller et al. 2013). Clients with dogs receiving any of these systemic therapies should ensure their pets' heartworm status is negative prior to treatment.

Client Education

The veterinary technician should discuss in detail the treatment plan with the owner. Correct bathing and dipping techniques, proper application of sprays and spot-on products, and correct administration of oral medications should be explained. Clients should receive a written copy of the treatment recommendations that they can refer to should any questions arise.

A follow-up examination should be scheduled with the veterinarian after four to six weeks of treatment. After six weeks of treatment, clinical signs have often resolved and microscopic evaluation for the presence of mites is usually negative. At the recheck appointment the veterinary technician should ask the owner to describe the treatment they have been doing, and determine if treatment recommendations were followed. The patient's degree of pruritus and any other clinical signs noticed by the owner should be recorded. The patient should be carefully examined for any signs of continued infestation, such as dry scale, papules, crusts, or alopecia. If mites were found previously or if clinical signs are persisting, flea combing, acetate tape preparations, superficial skin scrapings, or any combination of these diagnostic tests should be performed to search for *Cheyletiella* mites. Ideally, treatment is continued for two to four weeks past resolution of clinical signs and negative microscopic evaluation for mites. If infestation is continuing, careful questioning of the client is necessary to determine if the patient, all in-contact animals, and the environment are being treated adequately.

Conclusion

Cheyletiellosis is an important differential diagnosis for patients presenting with scale, papules, and pruritus. The disease poses a diagnostic challenge when asymptomatic carriers are involved and when mites are not found on the patient. Historical information regarding contact with other animals, presence of other affected pets or humans in the household, and flea control products used on pets and in the environment can help rule cheyletiellosis in or out as a differential. In some cases, only a failure to respond to miticidal therapy can exclude cheyletiellosis from the differential list. Eliminating an infestation can be a complicated process, especially in a multiple-pet household with a severe infestation. A thorough explanation of the mite life cycle as well as the entire treatment process will greatly increase the chances of a successful outcome.

References

Burrows, A. (2009). Avermectins in Dermatology. In: *Current Veterinary Therapy XIV* (eds. J.D. Bonagura and D.C. Twedt), 390–394. Philadelphia, PA: Saunders.

Chailleux, N. and Paradis, M. (2002). Efficacy of selamectin in the treatment of naturally acquired cheyletiellosis in cats. *Canadian Veterinary Journal* 10: 767–770.

Curtis, C. and Paradis, M. (2003). Sarcoptic mange, cheyletiellosis and trombiculosis. In: *BSAVA Manual of Small Animal Dermatology*, 2e (eds. A.P. Foster and C.S. Foil), 146–152. British Small Animal Veterinary Association.

Ghubash, R. (2006). Parasitic miticidal therapy. *Topics in Companion Animal Medicine (formerly Clinical Technique in Small Animal Practice) Elsevier Saunders* 21 (3): 135–144.

Guaguere, E. (1999). Ectoparasitic skin diseases. In: *A practical guide to feline dermatology* (eds. E. Guaguere and P. Prelaud), 3–4. Merial.

Meredith, A. (2006). Dermatology of mammals: skin diseases and treatment of rabbits. In: *Skin Diseases of Exotic Pets* (ed. S. Paterson), 288–311. Oxford: Blackwell Science.

Miller, W.H., Griffin, C.E., and Campbell, K.L. (eds.) (2013). Parasitic skin diseases. In: *Muller & Kirk's Small Animal Dermatology*, 7e. St. Louis, MO: Elsevier/Mosby, Chapter 4.

Page, N., de Jaham, C., and Paradis, M. (2000). Observations on topical ivermectin in the treatment of otoacariosis, cheyletiellosis, and toxocariosis in cats. *Canadian Veterinary Journal* 41: 773–776.

Paradis, M. and Villeneuve, A. (1988). Efficacy of ivermectin against *Cheyletiella yasguri* infestation in dogs. *Canadian Veterinary Journal* 29: 633–635.

Paradis, M., Scott, D.W., and Villeneuve, A. (1990). Efficacy of ivermectin against *Cheyletiella blakei* infestation in cats. *Journal of the American Animal Hospital Association* 26: 125–128.

11

Canine Demodicosis

Kim Horne

Introduction

Demodicosis is a common parasitic skin disease of young dogs. The disease can be localized or generalized, and each type has specific prognostic and treatment recommendations. The generalized form of this disease can be severe and is categorized as either juvenile-onset or adult-onset. While it can be relatively easy to find the mites and make a diagnosis, the disease is often challenging to treat. Clinical improvement can be slow, frequent follow-up visits are needed, and the length of treatment required to reach parasitological cure can be long. The time and financial commitment required of owners can be substantial (Horne 2010).

Demodex canis is the mite most commonly found in cases of demodicosis (Figure 11.1). It is a fusiform, cigar-shaped normal inhabitant of the skin and ear canal, living in the hair follicles and occasionally in the sebaceous glands (Miller et al. 2013). *D. canis* has four life stages: a fusiform egg, a six-legged larva, an eight-legged nymph, and an eight-legged adult (Figure 11.2). Neonatal puppies acquire the mite from their dam shortly after birth while nursing. Demodicosis caused by *D. canis* is not contagious. The disease develops when the mite population increases to a point at which the immune response is triggered and clinical signs develop. The tendency to develop generalized demodicosis is hereditary. Other mites that have been identified from dogs with demodicosis include *Demodex injai* (a long-tailed mite; Figure 11.3) and *Demodex cornei* (a short-tailed mite; Figure 11.4). The initial differentiation of the three species was based on physical description, but more recent DNA analysis suggests they might all be morphological variants of *D. canis* (Rojas et al. 2012).

Demodicosis is seen more often in purebred dogs (Gortel 2006; Miller et al. 2013) and puppies. The most common breeds affected can vary by region and may be related to the practices of local breeders. Any young dog (18 months or less) with suggestive clinical signs should always have demodicosis included in their differential diagnosis and a skin scraping should be performed. The juvenile form of this disease typically starts before the dog reaches one year of age. Juvenile-onset generalized demodicosis is a hereditary disease thought to result from a T-lymphocyte defect specific for the mites. Intact dogs diagnosed with this disease should not be bred and should be spayed or neutered (Mueller et al. 2012). Other factors considered predisposing include poor nutrition, endoparasitism, and stress (including estrus and parturition).

Adult-onset demodicosis typically starts after four years of age and often is associated with an underlying condition such as neoplasia, hyperadrenocorticism, hypothyroidism, or treatment with immunosuppressive drugs (Miller et al. 2013). It is important to identify

Small Animal Dermatology for Technicians and Nurses, First Edition. Edited by Kim Horne, Marcia Schwassmann and Dawn Logas.
© 2020 John Wiley & Sons, Inc. Published 2020 by John Wiley & Sons, Inc.

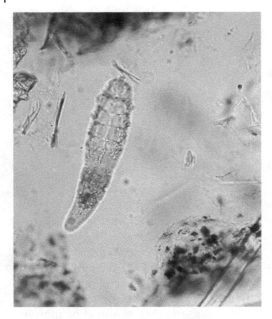

Figure 11.1 Skin scraping showing adult *Demodex canis* mite.

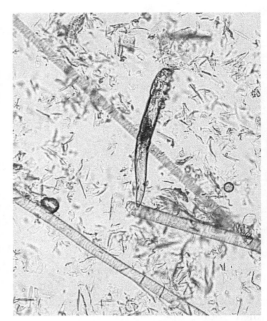

Figure 11.3 Skin scraping showing adult *Demodex injai* mite.

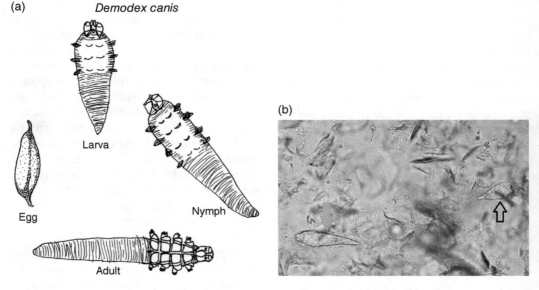

Figure 11.2 (a) The four life stages of *Demodex* mites. Egg: fusiform (spindle) shaped; larva: three pairs of short legs; nymph: four pairs of short legs; adult: four pairs of legs, defined chest detail. *Source:* Courtesy of Dr. Jane Gehr. (b) Skin scraping showing immature mite stages, egg (black arrow), and larva (blue arrow).

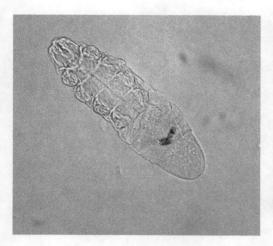

Figure 11.4 Skin scraping showing adult *Demodex cornei* mite.

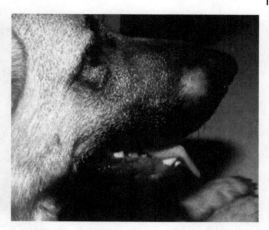

Figure 11.5 Patient with localized demodicosis, showing circular area of alopecia on the muzzle.

and treat any underlying disease and to minimize immunosuppressive drug therapy in these patients to increase chances of successful treatment of their demodicosis. In up to 50% of patients, the underlying disease may not be identified until well after treatment for the skin disease has been started (Miller et al. 2013).

Clinical Features

Localized demodicosis often presents with circular areas of alopecia with or without erythema, especially on the face and forelegs (Figure 11.5). Truncal involvement can also be seen. Pruritus is variable, but is usually not severe. There are no uniformly accepted criteria to differentiate localized from generalized forms of the disease. The committee that wrote the 2011 demodicosis treatment guidelines considers the disease localized if there are no more than four lesions with a diameter of up to 2.5 cm (Mueller et al. 2012). Most cases of localized demodicosis are seen in puppies between three to six months of age, and almost all of these spontaneously resolve without treatment. Demodectic otitis externa where the mites are found only in the ear canals is a rare form of localized disease.

When more than four areas are affected, or when an entire region of the body is involved (including two or more feet), the disease is considered generalized (Gortel 2006; Miller et al. 2013) (Figure 11.6). Bacterial pyoderma often accompanies generalized demodicosis. Pruritus may or may not be present, and is typically absent unless secondary infections develop. Patches of alopecia, erythema, scaling, comedones, papules, and pustules may be seen early in the disease. More chronic cases may also show hyperpigmentation, lichenification, severe crusting, furuncles, and draining tracts (Figures 11.7 and 11.8). Patients with demodectic pododermatitis can be especially pruritic and painful.

Peripheral lymphadenopathy may be noted and systemic signs such as fever, depression, and anorexia can occur if secondary bacterial infection is severe (Hnilica and Patterson 2017). Before the development of effective miticidal therapy, this disease was often fatal due to eventual bacterial sepsis.

D. cornei produces clinical disease identical to *D. canis* and mixed infestations may be found. *D. injai* has been associated with two clinically distinct syndromes, a greasy, erythematous, and pruritic dorsal truncal dermatitis and a severely pruritic facial dermatitis. Terriers, particularly West Highland white terriers and shih tzus, are predisposed. Mite numbers are typically low

(a)

(b)

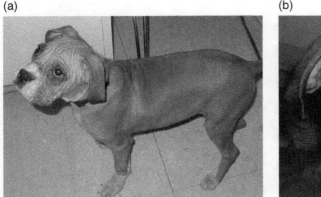
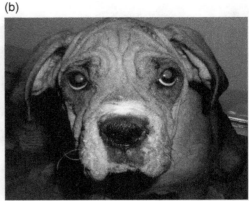

Figure 11.6 (a) Patient with juvenile-onset generalized demodicosis, showing entire body region (head) affected. (b) Closer view of erythema and alopecia on face.

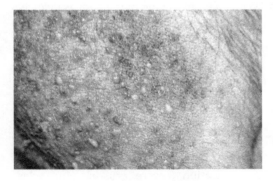

Figure 11.7 Pustules and comedones on a dog with demodicosis and secondary superficial pyoderma.

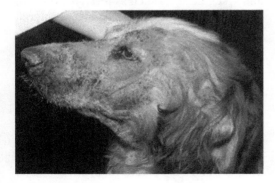

Figure 11.8 Patient with adult-onset generalized demodicosis, showing severe erythema, lichenification, and crusting.

in these cases (Hnilica and Patterson 2017; Koch et al. 2012; Miller et al. 2013).

Diagnostic Tests

Multiple deep skin scrapings are the most reliable method to diagnose demodicosis. *Demodex canis* is the species identified most often, but *D. injai and D. cornei* may also be seen. Proper skin scraping technique is essential to find the mites. Microscope slides should be labeled with the site to be scraped and mineral oil is applied to the slide. It is important to either dip the scraping instrument (a dulled #10 scalpel blade or spatula) in mineral oil or to apply mineral oil directly onto the area being scraped to ensure the material collected sticks to the instrument. Squeezing the site is necessary to extrude the mites that are deep in the hair follicles up onto the skin surface. Scrape deep enough to get capillary bleeding, transfer scraped material to the mineral oil on the glass slide, apply coverslip, and examine microscopically. Lowering the microscope condenser to increase contrast will help with mite visualization. Record results from each site scraped, identifying the life stage (egg, larva, nymph, or adult) and number of mites found, or at least an estimated percentage of the stages present (Figure 11.9).

Although a trichogram is not as reliable as skin scrapings for the detection of demodex mites (Saridomichelakis et al. 2007), this

Date:_____

Skin Scraping Site:_____

    Eggs:_____

    Larvae:_____

    Nymphs:_____

    Adults (dead):_____

    Adults (alive):_____

Skin Scraping Site:_____

    Eggs:_____

    Larvae:_____

    Nymphs:_____

    Adults (dead):_____

    Adults (alive):_____

Skin Scraping Site:_____

    Eggs:_____

    Larvae:_____

    Nymphs:_____

    Adults (dead):_____

    Adults (alive):_____

Skin Scraping Site:_____

    Eggs:_____

    Larvae:_____

    Nymphs:_____

    Adults (dead):_____

    Adults (alive):_____

Figure 11.9 Example of how to record skin scraping results in patient's medical record.

procedure may be useful for areas such as interdigital spaces or periocular skin that are difficult to scrape or too painful to scrape without sedation (Figure 11.10). Mites trapped in follicular keratin may be seen (Miller et al. 2013). The trichogram is less sensitive than skin scrapings, so a negative test does not rule out a diagnosis of demodicosis. This method should only be used for the initial diagnostic test, not to monitor therapeutic progress.

When mite numbers are high, they may also be found on acetate tape impressions from the skin surface or in exudate from draining tracts (Mueller et al. 2012). Tape is applied to the site and the skin is squeezed. As the mites are extruded from the follicle, they will stick to the tape, which is then applied to mineral oil on the glass slide and examined microscopically. When purulent exudate is present, it can be applied to a glass slide and mixed with a small amount of mineral oil and examined for the presence of mites.

Skin biopsies are occasionally needed to make the diagnosis. If the index of suspicion for demodicosis is high and skin scrapings are negative, a punch biopsy would be recommended. This procedure may be necessary in patients that have chronic pododermatitis, patients with thick skin (Shar-Pei; Figure 11.11), or patients whose lesions have become fibrotic.

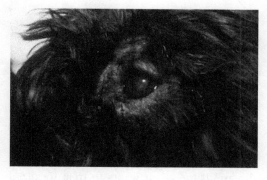

Figure 11.10 A trichogram may be needed in patients with periocular or interdigital involvement, such as this patient with localized demodicosis involving the skin around his eye.

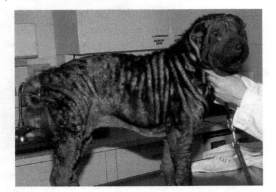

Figure 11.11 Because of their thick skin, if deep skin scrapings are negative, Shar-Peis may need a skin biopsy to be performed to confirm or rule out demodicosis.

Treatment

Treatment recommendations will vary depending on which form of the disease is present: localized, juvenile-onset generalized, or adult-onset generalized. All patients with demodicosis should not be treated with any immunosuppressive medications including glucocorticoids, if at all possible. Moreover, there are a number of drugs that should not be used concurrently with many of the miticidal therapies; obtaining a complete medication history is critical to prevent any adverse reactions in the dog. The patient's general health should always be assessed as part of the treatment for this disease and any problems should be corrected.

Localized Demodicosis

Patients with localized demodicosis often do not need to be treated, as most cases spontaneously resolve (Mueller 2004) within six to eight weeks (Miller et al. 2013). These dogs should not receive miticidal therapy unless their disease becomes generalized, and there is no evidence that early treatment of localized disease prevents progression to generalized disease. If the client wants to treat localized lesions, topical therapy with antibacterial products such as benzoyl peroxide gel can be used (Koch et al. 2012). Additional adjunctive

therapy may or may not be needed. These patients should be re-examined in one month to ensure that the lesions are resolving and not progressing to generalized disease.

Generalized Demodicosis

Most cases of generalized demodicosis require specific miticidal treatment as well as topical and/or systemic therapy for secondary bacterial/yeast infections. In middle-aged to older patients, determining the age at initial onset of disease can help differentiate chronic or relapsing juvenile-onset disease from true adult-onset disease. This is important, since the prognosis for adult-onset demodicosis is less favorable. Factors to consider when choosing therapy include patient history and breed, location and extent and severity of lesions, as well as the client's ability and willingness to be compliant with the recommended treatment.

For patients diagnosed with adult-onset demodicosis, a thorough search for an underlying cause should be undertaken. A comprehensive history and thorough physical exam should be performed and a minimum database including a complete blood count, chemistry profile, heartworm test, urinalysis, and fecal analysis collected. Specific testing to evaluate for hyperadrenocorticism and thyroid disease may also be indicated. In some cases chest radiographs and abdominal ultrasound may be recommended. In many cases an underlying disease is not found at the time of initial diagnosis. These patients should be monitored closely during treatment, since the underlying disease may manifest during the course of therapy. If the underlying condition cannot be resolved, the demodicosis will be more difficult to clear and long-term maintenance therapy may be required.

Amitraz

Amitraz (Mitaban®*, Zoetis, Parsipanny, NJ) is a sponge-on dip solution that should be applied at the veterinary hospital. It is currently the

---

*This product is not currently available in the USA

only product that is Food and Drug Administration (FDA) approved in the United States and Canada for treatment of demodicosis, and is licensed for use every 14 days at a concentration of 250 ppm (Miller et al. 2013). The solution is prepared immediately prior to use by diluting one bottle (10.6 ml) in 2 gal of warm water. The dip should be applied to the entire body, including both normal and affected skin, taking care to avoid getting dip into the eyes. Alternative therapies may be indicated in dogs with significant periocular involvement.

Dogs with medium to long hair should be clipped short before treatment is started to facilitate contact of the amitraz solution with the skin. Patients should be bathed with antibacterial shampoo prior to dipping. Bathing removes crusts, exudate, and scale from the skin surface and increases contact of the dip with the skin. The dog should be gently towel dried before the dip is applied to avoid further dilution of the amitraz. Once the patient is thoroughly saturated with solution, they should be allowed to air dry naturally. Make sure the patient is kept in a warm area until dry. The dog should not be bathed or be allowed to get wet or swim between treatments. This can pose a challenge for patients with demodectic pododermatitis, so alternative therapies may be recommended for these dogs. Protective clothing and gloves should be worn by the person applying the solution and the procedure should be performed in a well-ventilated area. Personnel who are diabetic, taking monoamine oxidase inhibitors, or have respiratory problems should not be involved with the dipping application.

Adverse effects reported with amitraz include allergic reactions (urticaria), skin irritation, bradycardia, hypotension, hypothermia, and hyperglycemia. Systemic reactions can be treated with the alpha-2 adrenergic antagonist yohimbine or atipamezole. Amitraz should not be used in patients with diabetes and those taking monoamine oxidase inhibitors or tricyclic antidepressants. Lethargy and sedation may occur, especially after the first treatment, and can last for 24–48 hours. Amitraz should be avoided in Chihuahuas and other toy breeds, as they may be more sensitive to this product (Koch 2017). The safety of amitraz in pregnant dogs or in puppies under four months of age has not been established.

Increasing the concentration of the dip solution and the frequency of its application can increase treatment success rates. Various protocols including a 500 ppm solution applied weekly and a 0.125% (1250 ppm) solution applied to alternating halves of the body daily have been used (Mueller 2004).

Amitraz has been used off-label for demodectic pododermatitis and demodectic otoacariasis as a 1:9 dilution in propylene glycol or mineral oil that is applied once to twice a week (Forsythe 2012).

Macrocyclic Lactones

Although treatment with the macrocyclic lactone products discussed here is not FDA approved in the United States, they are widely used because of their efficacy. Ivermectin, milbemycin, moxidectin, and doramectin have all been used successfully. Dogs must have a negative heartworm test before using these drugs and they can discontinue their regular heartworm preventative during this treatment. Adverse effects are uncommon and can include mydriasis, hypersalivation, vomiting, lethargy, ataxia, tremors, seizure, coma, and death (Geyer et al. 2007; Koch 2017). When treating growing young dogs, especially large-breed puppies, accurate weights should be obtained at each visit and dosages modified as needed.

Macrocyclic lactones are contraindicated in certain herding breeds (collies, Australian shepherds, and others) due to severe central nervous system side effects. These dogs have an increased incidence of a mutation in the *ABCB1-1 (MDR1)* gene that allows these drugs to accumulate in the brain. Genetic testing for this defect should be done in these breeds to determine if using the macrocyclic lactones is safe for a particular patient. More information about this gene test can be found at www.vcpl.vetmed.wsu.edu.

Ivermectin is a very effective therapy for generalized demodicosis (Mueller et al. 2012). The large animal injectable products are given orally once a day at doses ranging from 0.3 to 0.6 mg/kg/day. Neurotoxicity has been occasionally seen in non-herding breeds, so starting with a low dose that is gradually increased is recommended, for instance 0.05 mg/kg on day 1, 0.15 mg/kg on day 2, 0.2 mg/kg on day 3, 0.3 mg/kg on day 4, and so on (Mueller et al. 2012). Injectable ivermectin has a bitter taste, so mixing with something sweet can increase patient acceptance of the medication. Daily ivermectin should not be used together with other P-glycoprotein inhibitors – such as spinosad (Comfortis®, Elanco, Greenfield, IN), cyclosporine, itraconazole, ketoconazole – to avoid neurotoxic reactions (www.plumbsveterinarydrugs.com).

Daily milbemycin oxime (Interceptor®, Elanco, Greenfield, IN) is another very effective treatment for generalized demodicosis. The recommended dose is 1–2 mg/kg/day and it may be better tolerated and have a higher margin of safety than other macrocyclic lactones (Koch 2017). It should still be used with caution in dogs with the *ABCB1-1* gene mutation. This drug is labeled for use as a once-a-month heartworm preventative and daily use may be cost prohibitive, especially for larger dogs.

The large animal injectable form of moxidectin is another treatment that may be given orally at a dose of 0.2–0.5 mg/kg/day (Koch 2017). Efficacy is similar to daily ivermectin and gradually increasing dosages are also recommended for this drug. Adverse effects were seen more often with moxidectin than with ivermectin. Moxidectin is also available as a 2.5% topical solution together with imidacloprid – Advocate® (Bayer, Leverkusen, Germany) in the UK and Europe and Advantage Multi® (Bayer) in the United States. Weekly application of this product can be an effective therapy for milder cases of juvenile-onset generalized demodicosis (Mueller et al. 2012). It is labeled for this use in some countries outside the United States. It may be better tolerated than other avermectins and safer for dogs with the *ABCB1-1* mutation. It has also been prescribed at the recommended monthly dose for flea and heartworm prevention in patients prone to recurrent demodicosis in the hopes of preventing relapses (Koch 2017).

Doramectin is a long-acting avermectin that has also shown good efficacy for the treatment of generalized demodicosis. This drug may be administered either orally or injected subcutaneously once a week at a dosage of 0.6 mg/kg (Gortel 2006; Koch 2017).

Isoxazolines

The isoxazolines are the newest class of insecticides approved for flea and tick control in dogs. All four of these orally administered compounds have shown excellent efficacy and safety as treatment for generalized demodicosis. Rapid improvement in clinical signs and decreases in mite counts are seen.

Fluralaner (Bravecto®, Merck, Madison, NJ) is effective at the label-recommended dose of 25 mg/kg given with food every three months (Fourie et al. 2015). It may be used in dogs that are six months of age and older weighing 2 kg or more. There are no specific label warnings against using the drug in breeding, pregnant, or lactating dogs and it is safe to use in dogs with the *ABCB1-1* mutation. Caution is advised in dogs with seizures or neurological abnormalities. Adverse reactions are infrequent and include vomiting, decreased appetite, hypersalivation, diarrhea, and lethargy (www.plumbsveterinarydrugs.com).

Afoxolaner (NexGard®, Boehringer Ingelheim, Duluth, GA) is approved for use at 2.5 mg/kg every four weeks. The drug has been used every two to four weeks as treatment for demodicosis (Beugnet et al. 2016; Chavez 2016). It is labeled for use in dogs eight weeks of age or older and weighing 1.8 kg or more. Its safety in breeding, pregnant, or lactating dogs has not been evaluated and it should be used with caution in dogs with a history of seizures. Adverse reactions are rare and include vomiting, diarrhea, anorexia, lethargy, and dry flaky skin (www.plumbsveterinarydrugs.com).

Sarolaner (Simparica®, Zoetis) is approved for use in dogs six months of age or older and weighing 2 kg or more. Once a month administration at the label-approved dose of 2 mg/kg was effective for treatment of demodicosis (Becskei et al. 2018). It has not been evaluated for use in breeding, pregnant, or lactating dogs, but does appear to be safe in dogs with the *ABCB1-1* mutation. Adverse reactions are infrequent and include vomiting, diarrhea, and lethargy. Higher doses may cause neurological signs (tremors, ataxia, and seizures) (www.plumbsveterinarydrugs.com).

Lotilaner (Credelio®, Elanco) is approved for monthly use in dogs eight weeks of age or older and weighing 2 kg or more. It should be used with caution in dogs with seizures and safety in breeding, pregnant, or lactating dogs has not been established. Adverse effects are rare and include weight loss, increased blood urea nitrogen, polyuria, diarrhea, and vomiting (www.plumbsveterinarydrugs.com). The label dose of 20 mg/kg given with food once a month was effective for generalized demodicosis (Snyder et al. 2017).

Adjunctive Therapy

If the patient has secondary skin infections, the dog should be treated with the appropriate antibacterial and antifungal medications. These infections often increase the patient's pruritus level, and treating them will allow the patient to feel better faster. Medicated shampoos may also be beneficial, but should not be used between treatments when using topical miticidal products. Remember that glucocorticoids (even topical) and other immunosuppressive medications should be avoided in patients with demodicosis. Antihistamines (avoid monoamine oxidase inhibitors if using amitraz) or non-steroidal anti-inflammatory drugs can be used to manage pruritus or pain if needed (Mckeever 2009). All patients with superficial secondary skin infections should be treated with antimicrobials for at least one week after clinical resolution of symptoms. Dogs with deep bacterial infections will require longer therapy. Recheck appointments are necessary to monitor the response to antimicrobial treatment.

Evaluating the general health of the patient is an important part of the therapy for this disease. Proper nutrition, husbandry, treatment of concurrent diseases (such as endoparasites), and avoidance or reduction of stress such as elective surgery or boarding can all contribute to a more successful outcome. Dogs with adult-onset demodicosis should be evaluated for underlying diseases and these diseases must be treated.

Patient Monitoring

Patients should be rechecked frequently during therapy, initially every two to four weeks (Miller et al. 2013) and then potentially less often (every four to six weeks), depending on the degree of improvement seen. Each exam should include a physical examination and deep skin scrapings of three to five severely affected areas (Mueller et al. 2012). Scrape the same sites at each visit as well as any new lesions. Record the results and compare them to the previous visit. Successful treatment is indicated by decreased numbers of adult mites with each subsequent visit, including a higher percentage of dead mites compared to live mites. Ideally at the first recheck, few if any immature stages of the mites are observed. These results are a good indication that the treatment is efficacious and the owners are being compliant.

Clients may need to be reminded not to stop therapy prematurely, since dogs may look clinically normal even when mites are still present. Treatment is continued until two consecutive negative skin scrapings are obtained. Negative means not even one partial mite is observed on the skin scrapings. Therapy is then continued for one month after the second set of negative skin scrapings are obtained (Mueller et al. 2012).

The veterinarian may recommend having the patient return every three to four months for rechecks throughout the first year of remission. At these visits, the previously scraped areas are rescraped (the hair will need to be clipped to get a good scraping). Alternatively, the client can observe their dog closely for any evidence of relapse and bring the dog in if this occurs. The patient is finally considered cured after one year with no recurrence of disease.

Client Education

Dogs can show significant clinical improvement well before negative skin scrapings are attained. If clients are not made aware of this, they may stop treatment prematurely, which will cause the patient to relapse because mites are still present. Frequent communication with clients to answer any questions and offer reassurance throughout the treatment process is helpful. Providing written information about the disease, its treatment, and length of therapy required to reach parasitological cure will increase the chances of successful treatment. Encouragement to the client when even small achievements are reached is appreciated.

The client must understand and accept the challenges of treatment. The reported cure rate for juvenile-onset generalized demodicosis is 70–80%, up to near 90% with intense treatment, but this can take 6–12 months of miticidal therapy (Miller et al. 2013). Patients with pododemodicosis/demodectic pododermatitis or those diagnosed with adult-onset demodicosis carry a poorer prognosis. Some patients may never reach parasitological cure and will require some type of ongoing therapy to keep mite numbers low enough to prevent the return of clinical signs. The isoxazolines are showing great promise for making demodicosis much easier and less costly to treat.

If the patient is intact, spaying or neutering is recommended, as juvenile-onset generalized demodicosis is hereditary. Many clinicians will refuse to treat patients if owners intend to breed them.

Conclusion

Generalized demodicosis can be a severe skin disease, but newer therapeutic options are making successful treatment more attainable. The technician's role in collecting a thorough history, performing skin scrapings accurately, and providing good client education regarding this disease will contribute to early detection and treatment. The technician's involvement with required follow-up visits and client support throughout the lengthy treatment period will help to achieve a positive outcome in these difficult cases.

References

Becskei, C., Cuppens, O., and Mahabir, S.P. (2018). Efficacy and safety of sarolaner against generalized demodicosis in dogs in European countries: a non-inferiority study. *Veterinary Dermatology* 29: 203–e72.

Beugnet, F., Halos, L., Larsen, D., and de Vos, C. (2016). Efficacy of oral afoxolaner for the treatment of canine generalized demodicosis. *Parasite* 23: 14.

Chavez, F. (2016). Case report of afoxolaner treatment for canine demodicosis in four dogs naturally infected with *Demodex canis*. *International Journal of Applied Research in Veterinary Medicine* 14 (2): 123–127.

Forsythe, P.J. (2012). Demodicosis. In: *BSAVA Manual of Canine and Feline Dermatology*, 3e (eds. H.A. Jackson and R. Marsella), 164–172. Gloucester: BSAVA.

Fourie, J.J., Liebenberg, J.E., Horak, I.G. et al. (2015). Efficacy of orally administered fluralaner (Bravecto™) or topically applied imidacloprid/moxidectin (Advocate®) against generalized demodicosis in dogs. *Parasites & Vectors* 8: 187.

Geyer, J., Klintzsch, S., Meerkamp, K. et al. (2007). Detection of the *nt230(del4) MDR1* mutation in white Swiss shepherd dogs: case reports of doramectin toxicosis, breed disposition, and microsatellite analysis. *Journal of Veterinary Pharmacology and Therapeutics* 30 (5): 482–485.

Gortel, K. (2006). Update on canine demodicosis. *Veterinary Clinics of North America: Small Animal Practice* 36 (1): 229–241.

Hnilica, K.A. and Patterson, A.P. (2017). *Small Animal Dermatology a Color Atlas and Therapeutic Guide*, 4e, 135–145. St. Louis, MO: Elsevier.

Horne, KL (2010). Canine demodicosis. *Veterinary Technician* March: E1–E6. http://vetfolio-vetstreet.s3.amazonaws.com/mmah/ce/551d03e8414491b97d7edba24d29aa/fileVT0310_pr_horneCE.pdf (accessed May 2019).

Koch, S.N. (2017). Updates on the management of canine demodicosis. *Today's Veterinary Practice* 7 (1): 77–85.

Koch, S.N., Torres, S.M.F., and Plumb, D.C. (2012). *Canine and Feline Dermatology Drug Handbook*, 1e. Ames, IA: Wiley Blackwell.

Mckeever, N. (2009). *Harvey: Skin Diseases of the Dog and Cat*. London: Manson Publishing.

Miller, W.H., Griffin, C.E., and Campbell, K.L. (2013). *Muller & Kirk's Small Animal Dermatology*, 7e, 304–313. St. Louis, MO: Elsevier/Mosby.

Mueller, R.S. (2004). Treatment protocols for demodicosis: an evidence-based review. *Veterinary Dermatology* 15 (2): 75–89.

Mueller, R.S., Bensignor, E., Ferrer, L. et al. (2012). Treatment of demodicosis in dogs: 2011 clinical practice guidelines. *Veterinary Dermatology* 23: 86–e21.

Rojas, M., Riazzo, C., Callejon, R. et al. (2012). Molecular study on the three morphotypes of Demodex mites (Acarina: Demodicidae) from dogs. *Parasitology Research* 111 (5): 2165–2172.

Saridomichelakis, M.N., Koutinas, A.F., Farmaki, R. et al. (2007). Relative sensitivity of hair pluckings and exudates microscopy for the diagnosis of canine demodicosis. *Veterinary Dermatology* 18 (2): 138–141.

Snyder, D.E., Wiseman, S., and Liebenberg, J.E. (2017). Efficacy of lotilaner (Credelio™), a novel oral isoxazoline against naturally occurring mange mite infestations in dogs caused by Demodex spp. *Parasites & Vectors* 10: 532.

Webliography

Plumb's Veterinary Drugs. www.plumbsveterinarydrugs.com (accessed June 2018).

Washington State University College of Veterinary Medicine Veterinary Clinical Pharmacology Laboratory. http://www.vcpl.vetmed.wsu.edu (accessed July 2017).

12

Feline Demodicosis
Kim Horne

Introduction

Demodicosis is being recognized more often in our feline patients and this disease can be difficult to manage. Cats can have either localized or generalized demodicosis and can be infected with *Demodex cati* (follicular demodicosis) or *Demodex gatoi* (surface or superficial demodicosis). *D. cati* is similar in appearance to *Demodex canis* (long, slender tail), lives in the hair follicles and sebaceous glands, and can be found in low numbers in healthy cats (Figure 12.1). The ova of *D. cati* are slimmer and more oval compared to the spindle-shaped ova of *D. canis*. The two other life stages (larvae, nymphs) of *D. cati* are also narrower than *D. canis*. This mite is not contagious. *D. gatoi* mites are shorter and wider with a stubby tail and are found within the stratum corneum. This mite is highly contagious. Additionally, a third as yet unnamed feline demodex mite has been identified. This unnamed mite resembles *D. gatoi*, but is larger and has some other anatomical differences (Miller et al. 2013). Although reports of this mite are uncommon, they have been found in cats with concurrent illnesses (Moriello et al. 2013).

Follicular Demodicosis (*D. cati*)

Clinical Features

Cats with localized demodicosis will often present with areas of alopecia and scaling around the head and neck – specifically the ear pinnae, chin, and periocular areas. Ceruminous otitis may also be caused by *D. cati*, and ear swabs should be obtained from cats with otic discharge and examined for mites (Griffin et al. 1993). Although the localized form appears to be rare, this disease carries a better prognosis and may spontaneously resolve without treatment (Miller et al. 2013; Guaguere and Prelaud 1999).

Cats with generalized demodicosis will often present with clinical signs that include alopecia, scaling, patchy erythema, hyperpigmentation, crusting, and ceruminous otic discharge – especially in feline immunodeficiency virus (FIV) positive cats (Miller et al. 2013). Areas affected include the head, neck, legs, and trunk (Figures 12.2 and 12.3). Some patients may present with a poor haircoat and greasy skin. Siamese and Burmese breeds may be predisposed (Guaguere and Prelaud 1999; Miller et al. 2013). These cats may or

Small Animal Dermatology for Technicians and Nurses, First Edition. Edited by Kim Horne,
Marcia Schwassmann and Dawn Logas.
© 2020 John Wiley & Sons, Inc. Published 2020 by John Wiley & Sons, Inc.

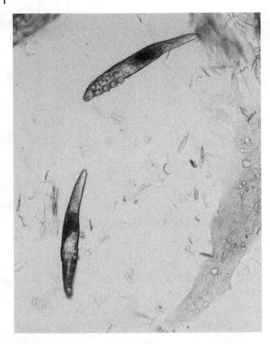

Figure 12.1 Skin scraping showing adult *Demodex cati* mites.

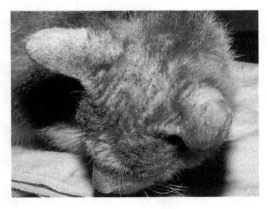

Figure 12.2 Cat with generalized demodicosis caused by *Demodex cati* showing close-up view of head region.

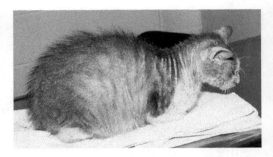

Figure 12.3 Whole body view of cat in Figure 12.2 showing clinical signs of alopecia, patchy erythema, scaling, and crusting. This patient was pruritic.

hyperadrenocorticism, toxoplasmosis, systemic lupus erythematosus, or squamous cell carcinoma in situ (Bowen's disease). These patients should have a thorough physical exam and complete medical history obtained, including current and previous medications – especially glucocorticoids. A minimum database consisting of a complete blood count, chemistry profile, urinalysis, fecal exam, FeLV test, and FIV test should be performed. The underlying disease may not always be identified when the demodicosis is first diagnosed.

Diagnostic Tests

Multiple deep skin scrapings to look for *D. cati* should be performed. Co-infection with *D. gatoi* or the unnamed mite has been reported (Miller et al. 2013).

Treatment

Localized demodicosis caused by *D. cati* can be self-limiting and resolve spontaneously. If treatment is needed, lime sulfur is usually effective for skin disease and otic preparations containing pyrethrins or amitraz in mineral oil (1 : 9) are effective for demodectic otitis (Miller et al. 2013).

Treatment for generalized demodicosis caused by *D. cati* is more problematic. Unless the underlying disease is found and managed, it will be difficult to cure the condition. The use of immunosuppressive medications such as glucocorticoids should be avoided. Lime sulfur dips are a safe and effective

may not be pruritic; however, when pruritic, the itching can be intense. *D. cati* typically affects cats that are middle aged or older. Generalized demodicosis in cats can be associated with immunosuppressive drug therapy or underlying immunosuppressive diseases such as feline leukemia virus (FeLV) infection, FIV infection, diabetes mellitus, therapy. Cats are dipped in a 2% solution once a week for a minimum of six weeks. The dip should cover the entire cat and be allowed to soak for at least five minutes. The patient should be allowed to drip dry in a warm environment. An Elizabethan collar might be needed to prevent the cat from licking itself and ingesting the lime sulfur, which can cause gastrointestinal upset (Beale 2012; Ghubash 2006). Treatment for *D. cati* mites should be continued until two negative skin scrapings taken four to six weeks apart are obtained.

Other treatment options for *D. cati* have been reported; however, use of these products is off label, and more information is needed about their efficacy. Weekly amitraz dips (0.0125–0.025%) have been used, but the risk of toxicity limits its usefulness. Other alternatives with easier administration or application are usually recommended (Beale 2012; Koch et al. 2012; Miller et al. 2013). Doramectin can be administered subcutaneously at a dosage of 400–600 mcg/kg. This treatment is repeated weekly until two negative skin scrapings taken four to six weeks apart are obtained, and then continued for an additional four weeks (Koch et al. 2012). Injectable ivermectin can be given orally (200–400 mcg/kg) every 24–48 hours until two negative skin scrapings taken four to six weeks apart are obtained, and then continued for an additional four weeks (Koch et al. 2012). Although ivermectin toxicosis is rare in cats, if seen it is usually in kittens within 1–12 hours after administration, and can be observed as abnormal behavior, lethargy, ataxia, weakness, apparent blindness, coma, and death (Miller et al. 2013).

Superficial/Surface Demodicosis (*D. gatoi*)

Clinical Features

D. gatoi is the short-bodied mite that inhabits the superficial layers of the skin (Figure 12.4). This species is contagious to other cats (Hnilica and Patterson 2017;

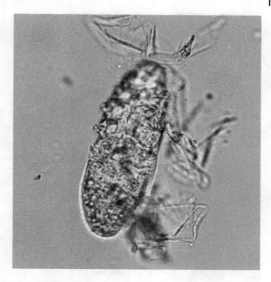

Figure 12.4 Skin scraping showing an adult *Demodex gatoi* mite.

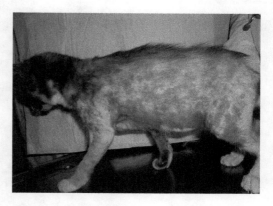

Figure 12.5 Cat with generalized demodicosis caused by *Demodex gatoi* showing clinical signs of alopecia.

Miller et al. 2013). Some cats are asymptomatic carriers of this mite and can be a source of infection for susceptible cats. Clinical signs, which can easily be mistaken for allergies, are the result of moderate to severe pruritus that is typical for this disease. Alopecia, erythema, hyperpigmentation, scaling, and excoriations may be seen (Figures 12.5 and 12.6). Pruritus may have a sudden onset and may not be responsive to steroids.

Superficial demodicosis may be found throughout North America, but is reported more commonly in the southern United

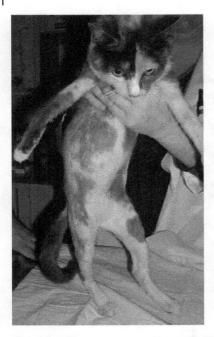

Figure 12.6 Same cat as in Figure 12.5, ventral view.

States, particularly in the Gulf Coast region (Beale and Morris 2009). This disease should be considered as a differential in any pruritic cat (Tater and Patterson 2008). Negative skin scrapings do not rule out superficial demodicosis; therefore a treatment trial may be warranted, especially as the clinical signs associated with *D. gatoi* can mimic allergic disease and self-induced alopecia.

Diagnostic Tests

Multiple superficial skin scrapings utilizing broad strokes to cover a large surface area should be obtained. Mites are more likely to be found in areas the cat is unable to groom well and are found more often in patients that are not pruritic. *D. gatoi* is easily overlooked on microscopy due to its small size and translucency. Using the 10x objective and lowering the condenser can increase contrast and make these mites easier to find. Other diagnostic tests that may identify these mites include trichograms, collection of surface debris with acetate tape strips, and fecal flotation examinations. If *D. gatoi* is not found on the pruritic patient, asymptomatic cats in the household should be checked, since they will not have removed mites from their skin surface by over-grooming (Beale 2012; Tater and Patterson 2008).

Treatment

Weekly 2% lime sulfur dips for a minimum of six to eight dips are also used to treat *D. gatoi* infestations. All cats in the household should be treated, since this demodex species is contagious. Use of a higher concentration of lime sulfur (3.1%) has also been reported (Ghubash 2006). A spot-on product containing 10% imidacloprid and 1% moxidectin (Advantage Multi® for cats, Bayer, Shawnee Mission, KS) showed good efficacy against *D. gatoi* when used weekly for 10 weeks in a multi-cat household (Short and Gram 2016). Since superficial demodicosis (*D. gatoi*) can be difficult to diagnose, a therapeutic trial may be needed to rule out the disease. The patient should be dipped with 2% lime sulfur once a week for three treatments. If improvement is seen, then the patient, along with any other cats in the household, should receive the full course of lime sulfur dips (Koch et al. 2012). If no significant improvement is noted after three weekly lime sulfur dips, then superficial demodicosis is unlikely. Weekly doses of Advantage Multi for cats can also be used for a therapeutic trial.

Other treatment options for *D. gatoi* include doramectin at 600 mcg/kg administered subcutaneously once a week and aqueous ivermectin at 200–300 mcg/kg administered orally once daily (Moriello 2013). However, due to the risk of neurotoxicity, ivermectin is not recommended over lime sulfur dip (Beale 2012; Tater and Patterson 2008).

Client Education

Clients need to be well informed regarding the underlying disease associations seen with *D. cati* as well as the contagious nature of *D. gatoi*.

Box 12.1 Tips for Owners Using Lime Sulfur Dip	
• Product can be drying, owner should wear gloves. • Use in a well-ventilated area. • Product is malodorous. • Product will stain light-colored fur (temporary). • Product will stain porous surfaces (cement or porcelain). • Product can change color (tarnish) jewelry. • Dilute product with warm water according to manufacturer's instructions and veterinarian recommendations. • Prepare immediately prior to use.	• Apply sterile eye lubricant prior to dip. • May be applied to cat in a bucket or sink, or clients may want to try a garden sprayer. • All areas should be saturated; may use rags, cotton balls, or gauze to wet facial area. • Do not rinse cat after application. • Allow product to drip dry naturally – do not towel dry or blow dry cat. • Use of an Elizabethan collar to prevent oral ingestion is recommended until the cat is dry. • May want to keep cat confined to a cat carrier in a warm location until cat is dry.

Treatment can be time consuming and frustrating, especially if the disease can only be controlled, but not cured. Although lime sulfur is a safe and effective product, it smells bad and dipping cats can be difficult. If owners are performing this treatment at home, providing a handout with helpful tips may improve compliance and prevent frustration (see Box 12.1). The imidacloprid/moxidectin topical spot-on product is much easier to apply than the lime sulfur dips and may become a more popular alternative. A treatment trial in pruritic cats with negative skin scrapings is often necessary to rule out *D. gatoi*. Doing so can save the clinician from making an incorrect diagnosis of allergic disease. Technicians play an important role in educating clients about the management of this disease to ensure that proper treatment and recheck recommendations are followed.

Conclusion

Although feline demodicosis is not a common diagnosis, it is an important disease to identify and treat if present. Because the clinical signs can be similar to other feline dermatoses, the veterinary technician should be familiar with the different presentations of this disease and feel comfortable performing the diagnostic tests required.

Having knowledge of the various mites that cause feline demodicosis and the different treatment recommendations will be beneficial for client communication and education. Keeping current as more information about this disease emerges, including diagnostic testing such as a polymerase chain reaction test (Frank et al. 2013) and new treatment options, will be an asset to your veterinarians and feline patients.

References

Beale, K. (2012). Feline demodicosis, a consideration in the itchy or overgrooming cat. *Journal of Feline Medicine and Surgery* 14: 209–213.

Beale, K.M and Morris, D.O (2009). Feline demodicosis. In: *Kirk's Current Veterinary Therapy*, 14e (eds. J. Bonagura and D. Twedt), 438–440. St Louis, MO: Elsevier.

Frank, L.A., Kania, S.A., Chung, K., and Brahmbhatt, R. (2013). A molecular technique for the detection and differentiation of *Demodex* mites on cats. *Veterinary Dermatology* 24 (3): 367–369.

Ghubash, R. (2006). Parasitic miticidal therapy, *Clinical Techniques in Small Animal Practice* 21(3): p. 139–140

Griffin, C.E., Kwochka, K.W., and MacDonald, J.M. (1993). *Current Veterinary*

Dermatology: The Science and Art of Therapy. St. Louis, MO: Mosby-Year Book.

Guaguere, E. and Prelaud, P. (1999). *A Practical Guide to Feline Dermatology*. Paris: Merial.

Hnilica, K.A. and Patterson, A.P. (2017). *Small Animal Dermatology: A Color Atlas and Therapeutic Guide*, 4e, p. 146. St. Louis, MO: Elsevier.

Koch, S.N., Torres, S.M.F., and Plumb, D.C. (2012). *Canine and Feline Dermatology Drug Handbook*, 1e. Ames, IA: Wiley Blackwell.

Miller, W.H., Griffin, C.E., and Campbell, K.L. (2013). *Muller and Kirk's Small Animal Dermatology*, 7e. St. Louis, MO: Elsevier.

Moriello, K.A. (2013). Chronic pruritus in a household of cats. *Clinician's Brief*, June. https://www.cliniciansbrief.com/article/chronic-pruritus-household-cats (accessed May 2019).

Moriello, K.A., Newbury, S., and Steinberg, H. (2013). Five observations of a third morphologically distinct feline *Demodex* mite. *Veterinary Dermatology* 24 (4): 460–462.

Short, J. and Gram, D. (2016). Successful treatment of *Demodex gatoi* with 10% imidacloprid/1% moxidectin. *Journal of the American Animal Hospital Association* 52 (1): 68–72.

Tater, K.C. and Patterson, A.C. (2008). Canine and feline demodicosis. *Veterinary Medicine* August: 444–461. http://veterinarymedicine.dvm360.com/canine-and-feline-demodicosis (accessed May 2019).

Glossary of Terms

Acantholytic cells keratinocytes (skin cells) that have lost their attachments to other keratinocytes, resulting in a rounded appearance on cytology and histopathology; often seen in pemphigus foliaceus, an auto-immune skin disease. See Figure 1.32

Acral lick dermatitis (acral lick granuloma, acral pruritic nodule, lick granuloma) a focal area of thickened, firm skin usually with surface erosion; typically found on a distal limb (acral); caused by excessive licking of the area. See Figures 2.17 and 7.15

Acral lick granuloma (acral lick dermatitis, acral pruritic nodule, lick granuloma) a focal area of thickened, firm skin usually with surface erosion; typically found on a distal limb (acral); caused by excessive licking of the area. See Figures 2.17 and 7.15

Acral pruritic nodule (acral lick dermatitis, acral lick granuloma, lick granuloma) a focal area of thickened, firm skin usually with surface erosion; typically found on a distal limb (acral); caused by excessive licking of the area. See Figures 2.17 and 7.15

Acute moist dermatitis (pyotraumatic dermatitis, hot spot) a localized area of moist, eroded, exudative, erythematous skin that usually results from self-trauma to the area. See Figure 7.16

Alopecia absence or lack of hair. See Figures 1.4, 1.33, 1.38, 1.44, 3.2, 5.5, 5.6, 5.8, 7.2, 7.5, 7.6, 7.8, 7.13, 7.14, 7.19, 7.22, 7.23, 8.5, 9.3, 9.5, 9.6, 11.5, 11.6, 12.3, 12.5, 12.6

Angioedema diffuse facial edema/swelling

Asymptomatic absence of signs or symptoms; used to refer to a disease that when present produces no outward signs or symptoms

Auto-immune disease disease that results from the immune system's attack on parts of its own body

Bulla (plural is bullae) a focal elevation of the superficial layers of the skin greater than 1 cm in diameter, filled with serum; also known as a blister

Callus a thickened and hardened area of skin that forms as the result of friction; usually over a bony prominence. See Figure 2.19

Cellulitis infection/inflammation of the skin and underlying soft tissue

Ceruminous pertaining to cerumen (ear wax). See Figure 4.9

Comedo (plural is comedones) a dilated, plugged hair follicle filled with sebum and epithelial debris; common term is a blackhead. See Figures 2.23, 11.7

Commensal term used to describe a relationship in which one organism derives benefit from another organism without causing harm, e.g. commensal bacteria are normally present on the skin surface

Crust a dried accumulation of inflammatory cells and/or epithelial

Small Animal Dermatology for Technicians and Nurses, First Edition. Edited by Kim Horne, Marcia Schwassmann and Dawn Logas.
© 2020 John Wiley & Sons, Inc. Published 2020 by John Wiley & Sons, Inc.

debris. See Figures 1.31, 1.33, 3.4, 5.6, 5.8, 7.10, 7.12, 7.13, 7.19, 7.22, 9.4–9.8, 11.8, 12.3

Cyst a closed cavity lined by a membrane, distinct from surrounding tissue; may contain liquid or fluid

Depigmentation loss of pigment

Dermatitis inflammation of the skin. See Figures 2.5, 3.1, 3.7, 3.8

Dermatopathologist/dermatohisto-pathologist a medical professional who specializes in the microscopic diagnosis of diseases of the skin

Dermatophyte a fungal organism capable of living on keratinized tissues, e.g. hair, skin, nails

Dermatophytosis infection of the hair, skin, or nails caused by dermatophytes

Dermatosis any disease or abnormal condition of the skin

Draining tracts (fistulous tracts) exudative openings on the skin surface that lead to a deeper focus of inflammation or infection. See Figure 2.20

Ectothrix refers to the formation of a sheath of fungal spores on the outside of the hair shaft. See Figure 5.10

Eosinophilic granuloma part of the eosinophilic granuloma complex in cats; a nodular lesion found most commonly on the caudal thighs or in the mouth

Eosinophilic granuloma complex term used to describe three types of skin lesions in cats: lip ulcers (indolent ulcers, rodent ulcers), eosinophilic plaques, and eosinophilic granulomas. See Figure 7.20

Eosinophilic plaque part of the eosinophilic granuloma complex in cats; a moist, erosive lesion found on the ventral abdomen and inguinal area. See Figure 6.11

Epidermal collarette a circular ring of crust that results from a ruptured pustule. See Figures 2.9, 7.4, 7.8

Erosion a lesion that results from the loss of the epidermal cell layers that stops above the basement membrane of the epidermis; will heal without scarring

Erythema (adj. erythematous) reddening of the skin. See Figures 1.33, 1.38, 3.3, 4.8, 5.5, 5.6, 7.2, 7.5–7.7, 7.11, 7.12, 7.19, 7.22, 8.4, 9.4, 9.5, 11.6, 11.8, 12.3

Erythroderma widespread erythema involving large areas of skin

Excoriation lesions that result from self-trauma to the skin. See Figures 1.14, 5.6, 7.3, 7.6, 7.21

Exudate fluid composed of serum and cells that leaks out of blood vessels from areas of inflammation or infection. See Figures 2.15 and 3.9

Fibrosis (adj. fibrotic) the development of scar tissue (fibrous connective tissue) in response to injury or trauma to tissue

Fissure a split in skin (usually thickened skin). See Figure 1.33

Fistula a draining tract

Fistulous tracts (draining tracts) exudative openings on the skin surface that lead to a deeper focus of inflammation or infection. See Figure 2.20

Follicular cast keratinaceous debris surrounding the base of a hair shaft

Folliculitis inflammation within the hair follicle

Fungal arthrospores/arthroconidia a type of fungal spore formed by the segmentation of fungal hyphae; found inside or surrounding hair shafts. See Figures 1.48 and 5.10

Fungal hyphae long, branching, filamentous structures produced by fungi as the main mode of growth; a mass of fungal hyphae is referred to as a mycelium. See Figure 5.16

Furuncle a focal, dome-shaped, often erythematous and painful lesion on the skin, usually associated with infection of a hair follicle that results in rupture of the follicle. See Figures 2.15 and 2.24

Furunculosis inflammation that has resulted in rupture of the hair follicle; fragments of hair shafts will be seen free in the dermis, usually surrounded by inflammatory cells. See Figures 2.14 and 2.18

Fusiform spindle shaped, tapered at both ends

Glycoprotein a protein with an attached carbohydrate group

Hirsutism excessive growth of hair. See Figure 7.25

Hive (wheal) a circumscribed, raised, erythematous area of skin

Hot spot (acute moist dermatitis, pyotraumatic dermatitis) a localized area of moist, eroded, exudative, erythematous skin that usually results from self-trauma to the area. See Figure 7.16

Hyperkeratosis an increase in the thickness of the stratum corneum (the most superficial layer of epidermal cells). See Figure 7.12

Hyperpigmentation increase in skin pigmentation, often the result of chronic inflammatory skin disease or endocrine abnormalities. See Figures 1.38, 2.10, 3.2, 3.4, 7.10, 7.12, 8.3

Hypersensitivity an exaggerated response of the immune system to a foreign substance; often used interchangeably with allergy

Hypertrophy the enlargement of a tissue which results from an increase in the size of its cells

Hypopigmentation decrease in skin pigmentation; can be the result of inflammatory skin lesions or immune-mediated skin diseases

Immune-mediated in the strictest sense refers to any process that involves the immune system; often used interchangeably with auto-immune, referring to when the immune system attacks parts of its own body

Immunotherapy the prevention or treatment of disease with substances that stimulate the immune response; immunotherapy for allergies involves injections of substances the patient is allergic to in order to decrease the patient's sensitivity to those substances

Impetigo a superficial skin infection usually seen in puppies; characterized by large pustules that are not centered on hair follicles; found usually on the ventral abdomen. See Figure 2.6

Indolent ulcer (lip ulcer, rodent ulcer) part of the eosinophilic granuloma complex in cats; a usually non-painful ulceration on the ventral surface of the upper lips. See Figure 8.6

Inflamed/inflammation a response by the immune system to infection or injury, characterized grossly by redness, heat, pain, swelling, and loss of function, and microscopically by dilation of capillaries which allows serum and white blood cells to move into the tissue

Interdigital between the digits

Intertrigo (skin fold dermatitis) inflammation/infection in a skin fold. See Figures 2.2–2.4

Intradermal within the layers of the skin

Keratin the primary structural protein that forms skin, hair, claws, feathers, and hooves

Keratolytic referring to the removal of the superficial layers of the epidermis

Kerion a nodular lesion caused by an exuberant inflammatory response of the immune system to a dermatophyte infection. See Figures 5.3 and 5.4

Lesion a term used to refer to any abnormality on the skin

Lichenification thickening of the skin with accompanying increased prominence of skin markings. See Figures 3.2, 3.4, 7.8–7.10, 8.3, 9.5, 9.6, 11.8

Lick granuloma (acral lick dermatitis, acral lick granuloma, acral pruritic nodule) a focal area of thickened, firm skin usually with surface erosion; typically found on a distal limb (acral); caused by excessive licking of the area. See Figures 2.17 and 7.15

Lip ulcer (indolent ulcer, rodent ulcer) part of the eosinophilic granuloma complex in cats; a usually non-painful ulceration on the ventral surface of the upper lips. See Figure 8.6

Lipophilic having a strong affinity for lipids (fats)

Mackenzie brush technique a method for obtaining a sample of hair and skin scale for fungal culture; involves brushing the entire haircoat with a sterile toothbrush

Macroconidium (singular)/macroconidia (plural) an asexual reproductive spore produced by a fungus; used to identify fungal species; larger than microconidia. See Figures 5.12, 5.14, 5.17

Macule flat area of discoloration up to 1 cm in diameter

Microbiome the microorganisms (or their collective genetic material) that inhabit a particular environment, e.g. a human or animal body

Microconidium (singular)/microconidia (plural) an asexual reproductive spore produced by a fungus; used to identify fungal species; smaller than macroconidia

Miliary dermatitis a descriptive term for skin lesions in cats that consist of multiple small crusted papules. See Figure 7.18

Moth-eaten a term used to describe a pattern of hair loss that consists of multifocal patchy alopecia; it resembles the multiple small holes found in clothing caused by moth larvae eating the fabric. See Figure 2.11

Mucocutaneous referring to the junction of mucous membranes and skin. See Figure 2.13

Multifocal having multiple areas of focus; e.g. multifocal alopecia means alopecia affecting several different areas, not just one

Nodule a solid circumscribed elevation of the skin greater than 1 cm in diameter caused by an infiltration of or proliferation of cells

Onychomycosis fungal infection of the nails

Otoacariasis/otodectic acariasis infestation of the ear canal with ear mites (*Otodectes cynotis*). See Figure 4.2

Ototoxic causing damage to the ear, specifically the inner ear (cochlea and auditory nerve)

Panniculitis inflammation of the subcutaneous fat, usually characterized by the formation of nodules and draining tracts

Papule a solid circumscribed elevation of the skin less than 1 cm in diameter caused by an infiltration of or proliferation of cells). See Figures 1.38, 7.1, 7.5, 7.6, 9.3

Paraneoplastic (in dermatology) refers to changes in the skin associated with the presence of a cancerous growth somewhere in the body but not due to presence of the neoplastic cells in the skin; e.g. paraneoplastic pemphigus foliaceus is a subtype of pemphigus foliaceus seen in association with neoplasia

Paronychia inflammation of the skin immediately around the nail base. See Figure 3.6

Pemphigus foliaceus an auto-immune skin disease characterized by auto-antibodies directed against desmosomes, the structures responsible for intercellular adhesion of keratinocytes; clinical signs include erythema, pustules, and crusting

Pinnal–pedal reflex a reflex used to indicate extreme pruritus in a canine patient, considered highly suggestive of scabies; consists of the patient attempting to scratch the ear with the hind leg when the ear pinna is rubbed

Plaque a solid, flat-topped, elevated lesion greater than 1 cm in diameter caused by an infiltration of or proliferation of cells. See Figure 2.21

Pododermatitis inflammation of the skin of the paws. See Figure 3.5

Porphyrin a dark red pigment consisting of four pyrrole rings connected by single carbon atoms; in dermatology used to describe the dark red/brown staining seen on fur/skin that results from salivary staining from licking or tear staining on the skin/fur ventral to the eyes. See Figures 3.5 and 8.1

Pruritus the sensation of itching

Pseudomycetoma a nodular lesion, often with ulceration and drainage, that results from infection of the deep dermis and the subcutaneous tissue with dermatophytes

Pulse dosing the administration of drugs in an intermittent, rather than continuous way; e.g. giving a drug daily for one week, then skipping one week, then repeating this pattern

Purulent consisting of pus. See Figures 4.10 and 7.12

Pustule a small, circumscribed elevation of skin that contains inflammatory cells. See Figures 1.38, 2.8, 11.7

Pyoderma (surface, superficial, deep) literally means "pus in the skin"; used to refer to bacterial infections of the skin. See Figure 2.7

Pyotraumatic dermatitis (acute moist dermatitis, hot spot) a localized area of moist, eroded, exudative, erythematous skin that usually results from self-trauma to the area. See Figure 2.1

Rodent ulcer (indolent ulcer) part of the eosinophilic granuloma complex in cats; a usually non-painful ulceration on the ventral surface of the upper lips. See Figure 8.6

Saprophyte a plant, fungus, or microorganism that lives on dead or decaying organic matter; term is used to distinguish non-pathogenic fungi from dermatophytes, e.g. growth of saprophytic fungi on dermatophyte test medium

Scale/scaling a thin piece of the most superficial layers of the skin, resembles a fish scale. See Figures 1.33, 1.42, 7.5, 9.6, 10.6, 10.7, 12.3

Scar fibrous tissue replacement that results from an injury to the tissue

Seborrhea oleosa descriptive term used to indicate greasy or oily, flaky skin

Signalment refers to the age, breed, and sex of the veterinary patient

Sinus an epithelialized draining tract connecting a body cavity to the skin surface

Stenosis narrowing; in dermatology is often used to describe the narrowing of the ear canal that results from swelling or tissue proliferation

T lymphocyte a type of lymphocyte (one of the white blood cells); in dermatology can be associated with skin cancer such as epitheliotropic cutaneous lymphoma

Thymoma a tumor originating from the epithelial cells of the thymus (a lymphoid organ in the chest of dogs and cats that produces T lymphocytes)

Trichography/trichogram microscopic examination of plucked hairs

Tumor a large solid lesion formed by an abnormal proliferation of cells

Turgidity the state of being swollen (turgid), particularly due to the accumulation of fluid

Ulcer (ulceration) loss of the entire epidermis including the basement membrane; exposes the dermis, heals with scarring. See Figures 7.10 and 7.14

Urticaria/hives/wheals multiple, erythematous, raised skin elevations filled with serum, usually pruritic

Vesicle a small, circumscribed skin elevation up to 1 cm in diameter containing serum; commonly known as a blister

Wheal (hive) a circumscribed, raised, erythematous area of skin

Wood's lamp an ultraviolet light source used as an aid in the diagnosis of dermatophytosis

Zoonosis a disease that can be transmitted from animals to humans

Index

Page numbers for figures are in *italics*, tables & boxes are **bold**

Small Animal Dermatology for Technicians and Nurses, First Edition. Edited by Kim Horne,
Marcia Schwassmann and Dawn Logas.
© 2020 John Wiley & Sons, Inc. Published 2020 by John Wiley & Sons, Inc.